A PROGRAMMED TEXT-WORKBOOK

THE LAST WORD IN MEDICAL TERMINOLOGY

MW01274995

ston

A PROGRAMMED TEXT-WORKBOOK

THE LAST WORD IN MEDICAL TERMINOLOGY

CAROL S. RUDLER-BARNETT, B.F.A.
Education Coordinator
St. Joseph Hospital
Mt. Clemens, Michigan

LUANN M. SUCKLEY, R.N., M.A.
Director of Patient Care Services
Spohn Hospital
Corpus Christi, Texas

Drawings by Carol S. Rudler-Barnett, B.F.A.

Little, Brown and Company, Boston/Toronto

ISBN 0-316-76094-3

Printed in the United States of America

MV NY

CONTENTS

PREFACE

DO YOU

Have the ability to analyze words?
Have the gift of memorization?

ARE YOU

Willing to look things up?
Now then, the task is to try to master a vocabulary rather than trying to learn a new tongue!

THE SUBJECT

MEDICAL TERMINOLOGY; BASIC ANATOMY AND PHYSIOLOGY; MEDICAL ABBREVIATIONS

HOW

By working your way through a programmed text-workbook you will be able to master the tests with an 80% accuracy.

The basis of this text is repetition. As you work you way through the text, you will be continually increasing your vocabulary but at the same time, you will be using what you have already learned so that it is not forgotten.

In the first several sections, terms may be used that are not actual medical terms (e.g., encephaloptosis = saggy brain). These are used strictly as a learning tool to demonstrate the potential flexibility of basic word structure.

This text is divided into 15 sections. Each section has an introduction, a body of information to be learned, a review test, and directions for what to do if your test score indicates that you need more practice. The answers to the review questions are in the back of the book.

Included along with this text is a cassette. You will be instructed when to use it for study. Frequently, you will find that you are directed to see the instructor for a specific test number. There will be designated times set aside for you to meet with the instructor for testing and/or questions you might have concerning your text. The programmed text should take from a minimum of five weeks to a maximum of ten weeks to complete.

In order to achieve the maximum benefit from this text, you must follow all instructions precisely.

C.S.R.B.
L.M.S.

ACKNOWLEDGMENTS

We wish to thank the administration of St. Joseph Hospital, Mt. Clemens, Michigan for the opportunity to pursue this endeavor, and extend our gratitude to the following people whose assistance in various capacities was invaluable: during the planning stages, Peter S. Suckley, Ed. S.; in the audio department, Daniel R. Ferguson, Audio-visual Technologist, and Cathy Pennington, B.A. Spec. Ed.; and for the typing, Sherry L. Arsenault.

THE LAST WORD IN MEDICAL TERMINOLOGY

BASIC WORD STRUCTURE

There are three steps in deciphering medical words.

1. Analyze the word's basic structure
2. Define the word by associating it with an anatomic system or disease process
3. Analyze pronunciation and spelling

First, one must learn basic word structure.

word root   Foundation of the word

EXAMPLE: *gastr* is a word root that means stomach

prefix   Word beginning

EXAMPLE: *epi*gastric—epi- is the prefix that means above

suffix   Word ending

EXAMPLE: gastro*cele*—-cele is the suffix that means protrusion

The medical term "epigastrocele" means protrusion of the upper stomach.

epi- (prefix) means above
gastr- (root) means stomach
-cele (suffix) means protrusion

combining vowel   A combining vowel, usually "o," links the word root to another word root or a suffix

EXAMPLE: gastrocele—"o" is the combining vowel linking a word root to a suffix

EXAMPLE: Gastrojejunocele—the first combining vowel links the two word roots, and the second links a word root to a suffix (the jejunum is the part of the bowel connected to the duodenum, which is the second part of the small intestine)

combining form   Combination of a word root with the combining vowel

EXAMPLE: *gastro*scopy—gastr- (root) + o (combining vowel) = gastro (combining form)

Adding the suffix "-scopy" gives us "gastroscopy," which means visualization of the stomach.

Some common combining forms and their meanings include

arthro Joint
carcino Cancer
cardio Heart
cerebro Brain
dermo Skin
entero Intestines
nephro Kidney
neuro Nerve
rhino Nose

Now can you analyze this word?

ELECTROCARDIOGRAM

Electr   o   cardi   o   gram
(root)   (combining   (root)   (combining   (suffix)
          vowel)   vowel)

Root: electr—electricity
Root: cardi—heart
Combining vowel: o
Suffix: gram—record or tracing

"Electrocardiogram" is the term for a recording of the electrical beat of the heart.

Summary

1. A word root is the foundation of the word (gastr).
2. A prefix is the word beginning (*epi*gastr).
3. A suffix is the word ending (gastro*cele*).
4. A combining vowel (usually an "o") links a root to another root or suffix (gastrocele).
5. A combining form is the word root with the combining vowel (gastro).

REVIEW

Now, let's assess what you know (circle correct answer).

1. What is a word root?
   a. a word beginning
   b. a word foundation
   c. a word ending

2. What is a prefix?
   a. a word beginning
   b. a word foundation
   c. a word ending

3. What is a suffix?
   a. a word beginning
   b. a word foundation
   c. a word ending

4. A combining vowel links
   a. a prefix to a suffix
   b. a prefix to a root
   c. a root to another root or suffix

5. Identify a combining form.
   a. cele
   b. rhino
   c. epi

Check your answers at the end of the book. If you missed more than one question, go back and study the preceding pages.

SUFFIXES

Suffixes are word endings that generally further describe or clarify the word root.

Suffix
-algia Pain
-cele Protrusion, hernia, or tumor
-centesis Puncture
-ectomy Excision, removal
-gram Recording, tracing
-itis Inflammation
-pexy Fixation, suspension
-scopy Visualization, inspection
-tomy Cutting into

A suffix changes the meaning of the word root. The following is an example of this (words with stars are not real medical terms):

Root/Suffix
gastr/algia Pain in the stomach
gastro/cele Protrusion of the stomach
gastro/centesis* Puncture into the stomach
gastro/cyte* Stomach cell
gastr/ectomy Removal of the stomach
gastro/gram* Recording of the stomach
gastr/itis Inflammation of the stomach
gastro/pexy Fixation of the stomach
gastro/scopy Visualization of the stomach
gastro/tomy Incision into the stomach

REVIEW

Identify each suffix and its meaning.

		Suffix	Meaning
1.	thoracentesis	_____	_____
2.	hepatectomy	_____	_____
3.	nephritis	_____	_____
4.	esophagoscopy	_____	_____
5.	cephalalgia	_____	_____

Check your answers at the end of the book. If you did not get 100% correct, review page 5.

On the following pages you will find 36 suffixes that you are required to learn. Each suffix has one or more meanings. Each suffix is used in an example or term. Each example or term is described. You are responsible for learning the suffixes and their meanings.

Suffixes	Meaning	Term	Definition
1. -algia	pain	arthralgia	joint pain
		neuralgia	nerve pain
2.* -ac	pertaining to	cardiac	referring to the heart
-al			
-ar (ary)	relating to	vascular	relating to the circulatory system
-ic	referring to		
-ory	denoting		
-ous		cutaneous	pertaining to the skin
3. -cele	hernia, tumor, protrusion	rectocele	herniation of vaginal wall into rectum or vaginal wall
		cystocele	hernia of the bladder
		hydrocele	serous tumor of the testis
		myelocele	protrusion of spinal cord through the vertebrae
4. -centesis	puncture	paracentesis	puncture of a cavity
		thoracentesis	aspiration of the pleural cavity
5. -cyte	cell	erythrocyte	red blood cell
6. -desis	binding, fixation	arthrodesis	surgical fixation of a joint
		tenodesis	fixation of a tendon to a bone

*These particular suffixes change word roots to adjectives and are frequently used when a prefix precedes the root. An example of this is epigastric.

7.	-ectasis	expansion, dilation	angiectasis	abnormal dilation of a blood vessel
			atelectasis	an airless, functionless lung; abnormal dilation of a bronchus or bronchi
8.	-ectomy	removal, excision	oophorectomy	removal of an ovary
			tonsillectomy	removal of tonsils
9.	-emia	blood condition	hyperglycemia	abnormally high blood sugar
			polycythemia	abnormal increase of red blood cells and hemoglobin in blood
10.	-genic	origin	bronchogenic	originating in the bronchi
11.	-genesis	forming, condition of, producing	osteogenesis	originating in the bones
			pathogenesis	producing disease
12.	-gram	tracing	bronchogram	x-ray of bronchus
13.	-graphy	process of, recording	arteriography	process of taking an x-ray film of arteries
14.	-iasis	condition, formation of, presence of	lithiasis	formation of stones
			cholelithiasis	presence of calculi in the gallbladder
			nephrolithiasis	stones present in the kidney
15.	-itis	inflammation	carditis	inflammation of the heart
			iritis	inflammation of the iris
			poliomyelitis	inflammation of the gray matter of the spinal cord

16.	-lithotomy	incision for removal of stones	cholelithotomy	incision into gallbladder for removal of stones
			nephrolithot-omy	incision into kidney for removal of stones
17.	-logy	study of	oncology	the study of tumors
			terminology	the study of terms
18.	-lysis	dissolution, breaking down, de-struction	hemolysis	breaking down of red blood cells
			myolysis	destruction of muscular tissue
19.	-malacia	softening	osteomalacia	softening of the bones
			splenomalacia	softening of the spleen

REVIEW

Match the following suffixes with their meanings:

1. -cele _____   a. breaking down

2. -cyte _____   b. incision for removal of stones

3. -ectomy _____   c. softening

4. -genic _____   d. origin

5. -iasis _____   e. protrusion

6. -lithotomy _____   f. removal, excision

7. -lysis _____   g. cell

8. -malacia _____   h. formation of

Check your answers at the end of the book. If you did not get 100% correct, review suffixes 1 through 19.

MORE SUFFIXES

Suffixes	Meaning	Term	Definition
20. -megaly	enlargement	acromegaly	enlargement of bones of the head and soft parts of extremities and face
		hepatomegaly	enlargement of the liver
		splenomegaly	enlargement of the spleen
21. -oid	like	fibroid	a tumor of fibrous tissue
		lipoid	fatlike
22. -oma	tumor	adenoma	glandular tumor
		carcinoma	malignant tumor of epithelial tissue
		sarcoma	malignant tumor of connective tissue
23. -ptosis	falling, drooping, saggy	gastroptosis	downward displacement of the stomach
		nephroptosis	downward displacement of the kidney
24. -raphy	suture	perineorrhaphy	suturing up a lacerated perineum
25. -osis	usually indicates an abnormal condition, disease	necrosis	dead tissue
		dermatosis	condition of the skin
26. -tomy	incision into	thoracotomy	incision into the chest
27. -pathy	disease	myelopathy	pathologic disorder of the spinal cord
		adenopathy	any glandular disease
		myopathy	any disease of a muscle
28. -pnea	breathing	eupnea	normal breathing
29. -penia	deficiency	leukopenia	abnormal decrease of leukocytes in the blood

handwritten annotations: ✗ (next to 23); -rhaphy (above 24); sp ✗ error (left margin near 24); -raphy circled; perineorrhaphy partially circled

30.	-pexy	suspension, fixation	hysteropexy	suspension of the uterus
			orchiopexy	fixation of an undescended testicle
31.	-plasty	surgical correction, plastic repair of	arthroplasty	surgical reconstruction of a joint
			hernioplasty	plastic repair of a hernia
32.	-rhexis	rupture	cardiorrhexis	rupture of the heart
33.	-scopy	inspection, visualization, examination	bronchoscopy	examination of the bronchi with an endoscope
			cystoscopy	inspection of the bladder with a cystoscope
34.	-spasm	involuntary contraction	bronchospasm	contraction of the bronchial muscles
35.	-stomy	creation of a more or less permanent opening	colostomy	creation of an opening into the colon through the abdominal wall
			cystostomy	creation of an opening into the urinary bladder through the abdominal wall
36.	-tripsy	crushing, friction	lithotripsy	crushing of calculi in the bladder or urethra
37.	-trophy	nourishment, development	mastatrophy	wasting away of the breast
			myotrophy	underdevelopment of the muscle

REVIEW

Match the following suffixes with their meanings:

1. -oma _e_   a. rupture

2. -ptosis _d_   b. breathing

3. -plasty _f_   c. disease

4. -scopy ____   d. creation of a more or less permanent opening

5. -rhexis ____   e. tumor

6. -pnea ____   f. visualization, inspection

7. -stomy ____   g. sagging, drooping

8. -pathy _c_   h. plastic repair of

Check your answers at the end of the book. If you did not get them all correct, review suffixes 20 through 37.

PREFIXES

Prefixes are word beginnings. Generally, prefixes describe the amount of or proximity or location relative to the word root.

Prefix
ante- Before
circum- Around
extra- Outside of
hypo- Below
intra- Within
multi- Many
post- Behind, after
sub- Under
trans- Through
tri- Three

A prefix gives the proximity to or amount of the word root. The following words are examples of this (words with stars are not real medical terms):

Prefix/Root
ante/gastric* Before the stomach
circum/gastric* Around the stomach
extra/gastric* Outside of the stomach
hypo/gastric Below the stomach
intra/gastric Within the stomach
multi/gastric* Many stomachs
post/gastric* Behind the stomach
sub/gastric* Under the stomach
trans/gastric* Through the stomach
tri/gastric* Three stomachs

REVIEW

Indicate each prefix and its meaning.

	Prefix	Meaning
1. circumocular	_____	_____
2. hypodermic	_____	_____
3. transurethral	_____	_____
4. postpartum	_____	_____
5. multiocular	_____	_____

Check your answers at the end of the book. If you did not get 100% correct, review p. 13.

On the following pages, you will find 59 prefixes you are responsible for knowing. Each prefix has one or more meanings. Each prefix is used in an example or term. Each example or term is described. You are responsible for knowing the prefixes and their meanings.

Prefix	Meaning	Term	Definition
1. ab-	from, away from	abnormal	away from the normal
		abduct	move a limb away from the body
2. ad-	to, near, toward, increase	adrenal	adjoining the kidney
		adduct	move a limb toward the body
3. ante-	before, forward, in front of	antepartum	before delivery
4. pre-		prenatal	before birth
5. pro-		prognosis	a forecast
6. anti-	against, opposite	antiseptic	agent used against bacteria
7. contra-		contralateral	opposite side
8. counter-		counterirritant	agent that irritates; normally acts against some other condition
9. circum-	around, about	circumoral	around the mouth
		circumocular	around the eye
10. peri-		pericardium	around the heart
11. co-	with, joined together, beside, along	coordinate	to work together
12. com-		compound	to mix or fuse together
13. con-		congenital	present at birth
14. sym-		symphysis	a growing together
15. syn-		synapse	joining of two neurons
16. dia-	through by, by means of, across	diagnosis	to find out the kind of disease
17. per-		percussion	a striking through
18. trans-		transurethral	through the urethra
19. di-	disengage, apart from, undo	diarthrosis	to separate a joint
20. dis-		discharge	to allow to leave

REVIEW

Match the following prefixes with their meanings:

1. ad- ____   a. around

2. anti- ____   b. through

3. co- ____   c. to, near, toward

4. per- ____   d. before

5. dis- ____   e. against

6. ab- ____   f. joined

7. pre- ____   g. apart from, undo

8. peri- ____   h. against

9. counter- ____   i. away from

Match the following suffixes with their meanings:

1. -desis ____   a. rupture

2. -itis ____   b. fixation

3. -tomy ____   c. inflammation

4. -rhexis ____   d. incision into

5. -rhaphy ____   e. suture

Check your answers at the end of the book. If you missed more than three, review prefixes 1 through 20 and the suffixes.

MORE PREFIXES

Prefix	Meaning	Term	Definition
21. ec-	out from	ectopic	not in the normal place
22. ex-	out from	exhale	to breathe out
23. exo-	outside	exogenous	produced outside
24. extra-	outside	extra-articular	outside a joint
25. endo-	within	endometrium	mucous membranes within the uterus
26. ento-	within	entocyte	cell contents
27. intra-	within	intravenous	within the vein
28. epi-	on, upon, above, in addition to	epigastric	upper part of the stomach
29. infra-	under	infrapatellar	under the kneecap
30. hypo-	beneath	hypodermic	under the skin
31. sub-	below, deficient	subclavian	under the clavicle
32. inter-	between	intercostal	between the ribs
33. intro-	into, in	introflexion	bending into
34. para-	near, past, beyond, beside	paravertebral	beside the vertebra
35. post-	behind, after	postoperative	after an operation
36. re-	back, back again	reactive relapse	to make active again a slipping back
37. retro-	backward, back of	retroflexion	bending backward
38. super-	excess, beyond, above,	supersecretion	an excess of any secretion
39. supra-	superior	suprapubic	above the pubic bone
40. tachy-	rapid	tachycardia	rapid heartbeat
41. ultra-	beyond, excess	ultrasonic	beyond the normal hearing range

REVIEW

Match the following prefixes with their meanings:

1. hypo- ___	a. rapid
2. inter- ___	b. out from
3. ec- ___	c. into, in
4. re- ___	d. back, back again
5. post- ___	e. on, above
6. extra- ___	f. behind, after
7. intro- ___	g. below, deficient
8. sub- ___	h. between
9. epi- ___	i. outside
10. tachy-___	j. beneath

Match the following suffixes with their meanings:

1. -spasm ___	a. like
2. -trophy ___	b. plastic repair
3. -oid___	c. nourishment
4. -plasty ___	d. involuntary contraction
5. -megaly ___	e. enlargement

Check your answers at the end of the book. If you missed more than three, review prefixes 21 through 42 and the suffixes.

MORE PREFIXES

Prefix	Meaning	Term	Definition
42. a-	without	apnea	without breath
43. an-	not	anesthetic	without sensation
44. bi-	both, two	bilateral	affecting two sides
45. tri-	three	tricellular	three-celled
46. quad-	four	quadriceps femoris	four combined muscles in thigh
47. tetra-	four	tetralogy of Fallot	an anomaly of the heart, having four features
		tetrad	group with four things in common
48. demi-	half	demilunar	a half-moon formation
49. semi-	half	semiconscious	half or part conscious
50. hemi-	half	hemiplegia	half paralyzed (paralysis on one side)
51. equi-	equal	equivalent	equal in power
		equilibrium	equal balance
52. multi-	many	multiform	many forms
		multipara	a woman who has borne more than one child
53. poly-	many	polycystic	many cysts
		polychromatic	many colored
54. super-	more, too	supernumerary	more than the normal number
55. per-	many	pertussis	excessive coughing
56. hyper-	excessive	hypertrophy	excessive growth
57. extra-	beyond	extrasystole	an additional contraction of the heart
58. sub-	less than (deficient)	submerge	under water
59. hypo-	below	hypotension	lower than normal blood pressure
		hypodermic	under the skin

REVIEW

Match the following prefixes with their meanings:

1. ultra- ___   a. many
2. bi- ___   b. four
3. equi- ___   c. half
4. hyper- ___   d. both, two
5. sub- ___   e. beyond, excess
6. quad- ___   f. equal
7. poly- ___   g. excessive
8. semi- ___   h. less than, deficient

Match the following suffixes with their meanings:

1. -algia ___   a. softening
2. -osis ___   b. recording, process of
3. -graphy ___   c. abnormal condition
4. -malacia ___   d. pain
5. -cyte ___   e. cell

Check your answers at the end of the book. If you missed more than three, review the prefixes and suffixes.

GO TO THE INSTRUCTOR TO TAKE TEST NUMBER 1 BEFORE GOING ON TO SECTION 4. YOU MUST ACHIEVE 80% MASTERY TO PASS. THE TEST WILL COVER PREFIXES AND SUFFIXES.

SECTION
4

WORD ROOTS

A word root is the foundation of the word. A word root names the subject.

EXAMPLE: myopathy

Myo is a word root meaning muscle. Muscle is the subject. Therefore, the word has something to do with muscles. *Pathy* is a suffix meaning disease. The word "myopathy" must then mean "disease of the muscle."

There are two illustrations showing word roots you are to learn. Start with Figure 1. Be very careful to learn to spell these word roots correctly. If a word is spelled wrong, you will not get credit for knowing it!

Many words sound the same but have different meanings.

EXAMPLE: ileum is part of the small intestine
ilium is part of the pelvis or hip

It is not only necessary to spell the word correctly, but also to say the word correctly. Play tape side A; the words shown on Figures 1 and 2 will be pronounced for you. When the root is pronounced, repeat it out loud; the word will then be pronounced a second time. You should also pronounce the word again. Stop the tape when the speaker says stop.

Only the words on Figure 1 will be pronounced before you will be told to stop. Stop before going on to Figure 2. It will also be helpful for you to write the word as it is pronounced to help you learn how to spell it. A work page is provided.

Now begin.

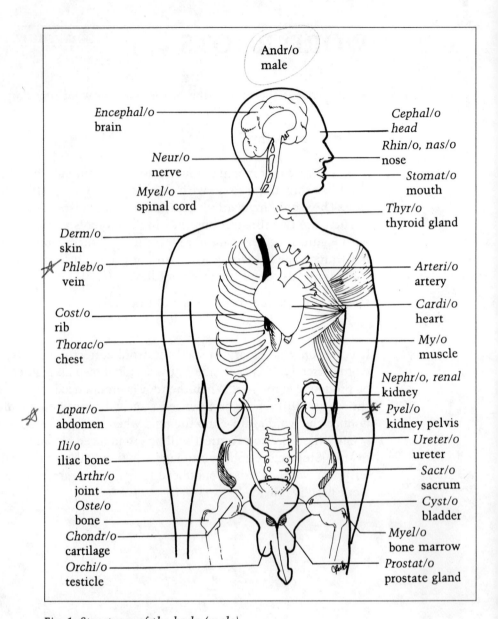

Fig. 1. Structures of the body (male)

WORKPAGE

Roots Combining
Combining vowel Forms
(o) added:

Andro - male
Encephalo - brain
Cephalo - head
Rhino - naso - nose
Neuro - nerve
Stomato - mouth
✗ Myelo - spinal cord
Thyro - thyroid gland
Dermo - skin
Phlebo - vein
Arterio - artery
Cardio - heart
✗ Costo - rib
Thoraco - chest
Myo - muscle
Nephro - Renal - Kidney
✗ Laparo - Abdomen
✗ Pyelo - Kidney Pelvis
Utero Uretero - ureter
Illio - iliac bone
Sacro - Sacrum
✗ Cysto - bladder
Arthro - Joint
Osteo - bone
Chondro - cartilage
orchio - testicle

✗ Myelo - bone marrow
Prostato - Prostate Gland.

2 meanings)

(28)

REVIEW

Give the meanings of the following word roots:

1. pyelo _____

2. thoraco _____

3. myelo _____

4. cephalo _____

5. thyro _____

6. cysto _____

7. orchi _____

Give the medical word root for each of the following:

1. abdomen _____

2. bone _____

3. artery _____

4. nose _____

5. muscle _____

6. prostate _____

7. mouth _____

Check your answers at the end of the book. If you missed more than one, go back and review Figure 1.

Now go on to Figure 2. Turn the tape on and begin where you stopped. Follow the same directions as previously stated for Figure 1.

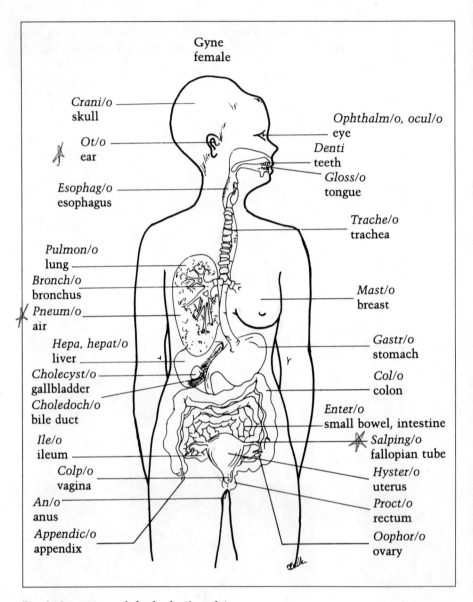

Fig. 2. Structures of the body (female)

WORKPAGE

No "o"

Gyne - Female

Cranio - Skull

8° Ophthalmo - oculo - eye

Oto - Ear

Denti - teeth

Glosso - tongue

Esophago - esophagus

Tracheo - trachea   (26)

Pulmono - lung

Broncho - bronchus

Masto - breast

Gastro - stomach

Pneumo - Air

Hepa, Hepato - liver

Cholecysto - gall bl.

Choledocho - bile duct

Colo - colon

Entero - Sm. bowel, intestine

Illeo - ileum

Salpingo - fallopian tube

Hystero - uterus

Procto - rectum

Oophoro - ovary

Colpo - vagina

Ano - anus

Appendico - appendix

REVIEW

Give the meaning of the following word roots:

1. denti _____

2. dermo _____

3. oophor _____

4. ileo _____

5. pneumo _____

6. hystero _____

7. broncho _____

8. oto _____

Give the medical word roots for the following:

1. skull _____

2. eye _____

3. tongue _____

4. breast _____

5. small bowel _____

6. gallbladder _____

7. appendix _____

8. anus _____

Check your answers at the end of the book. If you missed more than one, go back and review Figure 2.

COMMON RULES FOR THE ADDITION OF SUFFIXES
TO THE ENDS OF WORD ROOTS

vowels a, e, i, o, u (y)

consonants b, c, d, f, g, h, j, k, l, m, n, p, q, r, s, t, v, w, x, y, z

1. If the suffix begins with a *vowel*, drop the vowel of the root and add the suffix.

Root		Suffix		Word
hepato	+	*itis*	=	hepatitis
cholecysto	+	*ectomy*	=	cholecystectomy
nephro	+	*osis*	=	nephrosis
gastro	+	*optosis*	=	gastroptosis
neuro	+	*algia*	=	neuralgia

2. If the suffix begins with a consonant, add it to the word root in total.

Root		Suffix		Word
myo	+	pathy	=	myopathy
cardio	+	megaly	=	cardiomegaly
osteo	+	malacia	=	osteomalacia
thoraco	+	tomy	=	thoracotomy

3. There are always exceptions to the rule. Here is one of them: When adding the suffix *-rhaphy* or *-rhexis*, double the initial consonant before adding the suffix.

Root		Suffix		Word
arterio	+	rhexis	=	arteriorrhexis
orchio	+	rhaphy	=	orchiorrhaphy

You must remember that all of the above word roots are combining forms.

REVIEW

Add a suffix and give the definition of the entire word.

EXAMPLE: colo*tomy*—incision into the large bowel

1. tracheo _____   _____

2. broncho _____   _____

3. colpo _____   _____

4. cysto _____   _____

5. stomato _____   _____

6. hyster _____   _____

7. hepato _____   _____

8. denti _____   _____

9. oto _____   _____

It is possible to add many suffixes to a word root and *change the meaning of the word*. The following is an example of this. *Encephalo* is the word root. These words are pronounced for you on the tape (words with stars are not real medical terms).

encephalalgia   Pain in the head (brain)
encephalocele   Hernia of brain tissue
encephalocentesis*   Puncture into the brain
encephalocyte*   Brain cell
encephalectasis*   Abnormal expansion of the brain
encephalectomy*   Removal of all or part of the brain
encephalogram   X-ray of the brain
encephaliasis*   Condition of the brain
encephalitis   Inflammation of the brain
encephalolith   Calculi of the brain
encephalolysis*   Breakdown of brain tissue
encephalomalacia   Softening of brain tissue
encephalomegaly*   Enlargement of the brain
encephaloma   Tumor of the brain
encephaloptosis*   Saggy brain
encephalorrhaphy*   To suture torn brain
encephalosis*   Rotten brain tissue
encephalotomy   Incision into the brain
encephalopathy   Any disorder of the brain
encephalopexy*   Fix up, suture saggy brain
encephaloplasty*   Surgical correction of the brain
encephalorrhexis   Brain rupture
encephaloscopy   Inspection of the brain
encephalostomy*   Creation of an opening into the brain

The same thing can be done with prefixes by adding different prefixes to a root. *Thyro* means thyroid. *Fill in the meaning of the following words (words with stars are not real medical terms):*

1. prethyroid _____

2. circumthyroid* _____

3. transthyroid* _____

4. exothyroid* _____

5. endothyroid* _____

6. hypothyroid _____

7. parathyroid _____

8. suprathyroid* _____

9. multithyroid* _____

10. hyperthyroid _____

Check your answers at the end of the book. If you missed more than one, review the prefixes. Also, review Figures 1 and 2.

GO TO THE INSTRUCTOR AND TAKE TEST NUMBER 2 ON WORD ROOTS. YOU MUST ACHIEVE 80% MASTERY ON THIS TEST TO PASS.

exam Wed. 12th

REVIEW

Let's review what you have learned so far.

1. What are the three basic word structures?
   a.
   b.
   c.

2. Underline the combining form and circle the combining vowel.

   BRONCHOCELE

3. Suffixes describe or clarify word roots. ____True ____False

4. Prefixes state amount or proximity. ____True ____False

5. Indicate "P" for prefix or "S" for suffix.

   a. peri ____   f. intro ____

   b. itis ____   g. plasty ____

   c. anti ____   h. extra ____

   d. hemi ____   i. hypo ____

   e. desis ____   j. emia ____

6. A word root is the word foundation. Give the meaning of these word roots:

   a. costo _____

   b. cardio _____

   c. neuro _____

   d. hepa _____

7. Translate the following into word roots:

   a. ovary _____

   b. ear _____

   c. skin _____

   d. fallopian tube _____

8. There are two *general* rules for adding suffixes to word roots. What are they?
   a.
   b.

9. What is an exception to the rule?

Check your answers at the end of the book. If you missed more than five, review Sections 1 through 5.

The following lesson uses the general rules for adding suffixes. Recall from memory the prefixes and suffixes you have already learned. Fill in each line with either the medical term or the definition of the term written.

At the end of this lesson, continue with your tape. The correct answers to this study exercise are on the tape.

If you have difficulty, consult Taber's Medical Dictionary.

otology _____

otomycosis _____

otopathy _____

otoplasty _____

_____ protrusion of part of the brain through the skull

craniectomy _____

craniology _____

_____ incision into the skull

cranioplasty _____

_____ any disease of the skull

_____ creation of an opening into the skull

tracheomalacia _____

_____ disease of the pharynx

oculomotor _____

_____ toothache

glossectomy _____

_____ originating in the bronchiole

_____ one of the larger passages conveying air to and within lungs

bronchiole _____

_____ paralysis of bronchial tubes

bronchocele _____

_____ puncture of a lung for drainage of a cyst or abcess

pneumonomycosis _____

gastroptosis _____

_____ plastic repair of the stomach

7

gastrosis _____

_____ pain in the colon

choledochostomy _____

choledocholithotripsy _____

_____ tumor of the liver

_____ any functional disorder of the liver

hepatopexy _____

_____ inflammation of the gallbladder

cholecystostomy _____

_____ surgical puncture into the intestine

enterocele _____

_____ fixation of an ovary

oophorectomy _____

_____ stones in the fallopian tube

salpingectomy _____

_____ a condition of the appendix

appendicectasis _____

_____ excision of the ileum

ileostomy _____

_____ instrument used for examining the rectum

proctotomy _____

proctoptosis _____

anoscopy _____

_____ dilation of vagina

colpopexy _____

colposcope _____

_____ formation of nasal calculi

rhinoscopy _____

rhinalgia _____

encephalolith _____

_____ specialist in diseases of the nervous system

left of *paralysis?* [37]

neuromalacia _____

_____ surgical repair of nerves

neurogenic _____

stomatoplasty _____

_____ any mouth disease

stomatitis _____

_____ paralysis of spinal origin

myelomalacia _____

_____ spinal cord protrusion

_____ study and science of veins and their diseases

phleborrhexis _____

phlebolithiasis _____

_____ inflammation of a vein

_____ downward displacement of the thyroid gland

thyrosis _____

_____ incision into the thyroid gland

_____ rupture of an artery

arteriopathy _____

_____ suture of an artery

costectomy _____

_____ pain in a rib or in the intercostal space

myoma _____

_____ any disease or abnormal condition of muscle

_____ muscular protrusion

cardiocentesis _____

cardiectasis _____

cardiolith _____

cardiovalvulitis _____

pyelotomy _____

_____ reparative operation on the renal pelvis

pyelopathy _____

thoracoscopy _____

thoracostomy _____

thoracotomy _____

_____ surgical attachment of a floating kidney

renopathy _____

nephritis _____

ureterolithotomy _____

_____ surgical repair of ureter

laparoscopy _____

_____ abdominal wall rupture

sacralgia _____

arthrodesis _____

_____ pain in a joint

ostemia _____

_____ a bony tumor

osteitis _____

costectomy _____

_____ calculi in the bladder

chondritis _____

_____ softening of cartilage

_____ inflammation of bone marrow

_____ suturing of an undescended testicle in the scrotum

orchialgia _____

orchidoptosis _____

_____ pain in the prostate

prostatitis _____

prostatomy _____

The answers are on your tape.

COMPOUND WORDS

Remember that combining vowels connect a root to another root or to a suffix. If there are two or more word roots in the term, the word is said to be compound.

Consider the following word:

CHOLEDOCHOENTEROSTOMY

root   combining   root   combining   suffix
       vowel   vowel

Root: *choledoch*—bile duct
Root: *entero*—small intestine
Combining vowel: *o*
Suffix: *-stomy*

"Choledochoenterostomy" means to make a more or less permanent opening into the bile duct and small intestine.
   Medical terminology is made up of many compound words.

Translate the following compound words:

1. **salpingoureterostomy** _____

2. **neurodermatosis** _____

3. **nephroureterectomy** _____

4. **nephrocystitis** _____

5. **salpingo-oophorectomy** _____

6. **cholecystocolotomy** _____

Check your answers at the end of the book. Turn on the tape; the compound words will be pronounced for you. Repeat each word after it is pronounced.

SEE THE INSTRUCTOR FOR TEST NUMBER 3, WHICH INCLUDES PREFIXES, SUFFIXES, WORD ROOTS, AND COMPOUND WORDS. YOU MUST ACHIEVE 80% MASTERY TO PASS.

BASIC ANATOMY AND PHYSIOLOGY

The body may be thought of as a house with four major rooms. The rooms are called *cavities* (Fig. 3). The four body cavities house all of the organs in the body. They are

1. Thoracic cavity
2. Abdominopelvic cavity
3. Cranial cavity
4. Spinal cavity

The following organs are found in the *thoracic cavity:* lungs, heart, great vessels, trachea, and esophagus. The cavity is lined with a membrane called the pleura.

In the *abdominopelvic cavity,* the largest in the body, are found the following organs: stomach, large and small intestines, liver, gallbladder, pancreas, spleen, kidneys, ureters, and reproductive organs. The cavity is encased by a membrane called the peritoneum.

The *cranial cavity* is the space inside the skull that houses the brain. It is surrounded by three meningeal layers: the pia mater, the arachnoid membrane, and the dura mater.

The *spinal cavity* is the space that houses the spinal column. Like the brain, it is also surrounded by meninges.

The body is made up of eight systems (refer to the lists in Figure 3). A *system* comprises a group of organs that work together to perform a similar function. For example, in the circulatory system, the heart, blood vessels, and lymphatic vessels all work together to supply the body with nutrients and oxygen. The eight body systems are

1. Skeletal and muscular
2. Nervous
3. Circulatory
4. Digestive
5. Respiratory
6. Urinary
7. Reproductive
8. Endocrine

In Sections 7 through 11, we will present a basic introduction to all of the systems.

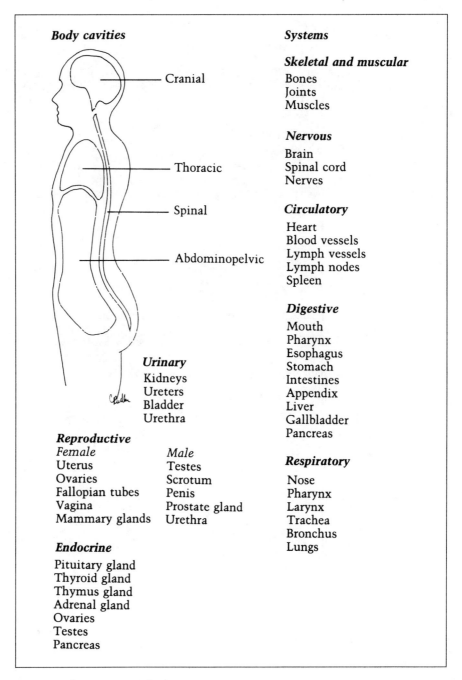

Fig. 3. Body cavities and systems

REVIEW

Answer the following questions:

1. The body is divided into cavities. Which of the following is not a cavity?
   a. spinal
   b. nervous
   c. cranial
   d. thoracic

2. Most of the organs of the body are found in the
   a. cranial cavity
   b. spinal cavity
   c. abdominopelvic cavity
   d. thoracic cavity

3. A body system is made up of a group of organs that work together to perform a similar function. ____ True ____ False

4. There are _____ body systems.

Check your answers at the end of the book. If you missed any questions, review pages 41 and 42.

The body is made up of structural units that build together to form the entire body. The *cell* is the smallest structural unit of all living things. Some living things are so simple that they are made up of just one cell; for example, germs consist of only one cell. Some living things are so complex that they consist of billions of cells—the humany body, for example.

Tissues are groups of like cells. For example, many muscle cells grouped together form muscle tissue. *Organs* are structures composed of several kinds of tissues that work together to perform a specific function. *Systems,* as discussed earlier, are groups of organs that work together to perform a specific function.

The medical terms that you are responsible for learning are presented in blocks of approximately fifteen terms. The following is the first block of terms you must learn. These terms are pronounced on your tape. Try to learn the words completely before going on to a new block of words. An asterisk indicates an easy association for learning.

Block 1

anomaly	chronic	energy	hereditary
benign	congenital	etiology	inguinal
brachial	cutaneous	foramen	loin
carcinoma	cytology	fossa	

anomaly (ă-nŏm′ăl-lē)   An irregularity; something out of the ordinary
benign (bĕ-nīn′)   Not recurrent; not cancerous
brachial (brā′kĭ-ăl)   Pertaining to the arm (*break the arm)
carcinoma (kăr″sĭ-nō′-mă)   Cancer; a malignant tumor
chronic (krŏn′ik)   Anything of long duration
congenital (kŏn-jĕn′ĭ-tăl)   Present at birth
cutaneous (kū-tā′nē-ŭs)   Pertaining to the skin (skin injections are given sub q, or subcutaneously, which means beneath the skin)
cytology (sī-tŏl′ō-jē)   Study of cells (cyte = cells; ology = study of)
energy (ĕn′ĕr-jē)   Capacity for a system to do work
etiology (ē″tĭ-ŏl′ō-jē)   Study of the causes of diseases
foramen (for-ā′mĕn)   Small opening
fossa (fŏs′ă)   Cavity or hollow
hereditary (he″red′i-tĕr-ē)   Transmission of characteristics from parent to child
inguinal (ĭng′gwĭ-năl)   Of the groin
loin (loyn)   Area of back between ribs and hip (*loin chop)

Practice writing and saying each word five times.

REVIEW

Match each term with its proper meaning.

1. cutaneous ____   a. area of back between ribs and hip

2. etiology ____   b. irregularity

3. foramen ____   c. pertaining to the skin

4. loin ____   d. small opening

5. anomaly ____   e. study of causes of diseases

Unscramble the following terms:

6. pertaining to the arm
   (lcbaiarh)   _____

7. of the groin
   (nginulai)   _____

8. malignant tumor
   (rmocainca)   _____

Check your answers at the end of the book. If you missed more than one, go back and review Block 1.

Block 2

Proceed to the next block of terms. The terms are pronounced on your tape.

lumbar	neoplasm	necrosis	sinus
involuntary	palliative	prognosis	stimulus
malignant	postmortem	ptosis	syndrome
meatus	moribund	sibling	

lumbar (lŭm'bar)   Of or near the loin
involuntary (in-vŏl'ŭn-tĕr"ē)   Not willed; no control over
malignant (mă-lĭg'nănt)   Deadly or cancerous
meatus (mē-ā'tŭs)   Passageway (*meet us at the passageway)
neoplasm (nē'ō-plăzm)   A new growth; a tumor
palliative (păl'ĭ-ă"tĭv)   Offering temporary relief
postmortem (pōst-mŏr'tĕm)   After death
moribund (mōr'ĭ-bŭnd)   In a dying condition
necrosis (nĕ-krō'sĭs)   Decay of tissue
prognosis (prŏg-nō'sĭs)   Forecast of the outcome of a disease
ptosis (tō'sĭs)   Dropping or drooping of an organ or part
sibling (sĭb'lĭng)   Children of same parents; brothers or sisters
sinus (sī'nŭs)   Cavity
stimulus (stĭm'ū-lŭs)   Agent that causes a change in the activity of a
      structure
syndrome (sĭn'drōm)   A set of symptoms that occur together

Practice writing and saying each term five times.

REVIEW

Match the terms to their proper meanings.

1. neoplasm _____   a. decay of tissue

2. necrosis _____   b. cavity

3. sinus _____   c. a new growth; a tumor

4. meatus _____   d. of or near the loins

5. lumbar _____   e. passageway

Circle the correct spelling and define each item.

6. PALIATIVE   PALLIATIVE   PALLIETIVE

_____

7. MORIBUND   MORRIBAND   MORIBOND

_____

8. SYNDROME   SINDROME   SYMDROME

_____

Are the following statements true or false?

9. An organ is a structure made up of several kinds of tissues that work toward a common goal. _____ True _____ False

10. Tissues are the smallest structural unit of all living things. _____ True _____ False

11. The thoracic cavity houses more organs than any other cavity. _____ True _____ False

Check your answers at the end of the book. If you missed any, go back and review Blocks 1 and 2.

ASK THE INSTRUCTOR FOR TEST NUMBER 4. YOU MUST ACHIEVE AT LEAST 80% MASTERY ON THIS TEST TO PASS. THE TEST WILL COVER SECTION 6.

SKELETAL AND MUSCULAR SYSTEMS

SKELETAL SYSTEM

The skeletal system has six functions.

1. Gives support
2. Gives shape
3. Protects inner organs and structures
4. Anchors muscles
5. Makes blood cells
6. Stores calcium

An infant is born with 350 bones. During growth, many of these bones fuse so that an adult has 206 bones (Fig. 4). Bones can be divided into two groups.

1. **Axial** These are the bones around the axis or middle of the body, including the ribs, breastbone, backbone, and skull. Axial bones form a protective shield around vulnerable organs. Axial bones form and protect the head and trunk.
2. **Appendicular** These bones attach to the axial bones and include the bones in the upper and lower extremities (arms and legs). Appendicular bones are levers for muscles.

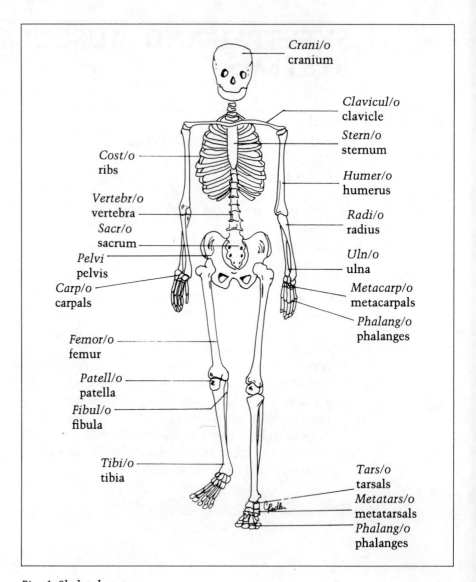

Fig. 4. Skeletal system

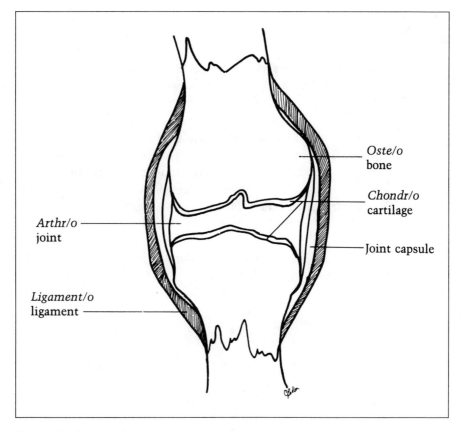

Fig. 5. A joint

How Bones Move

The places where two or more bones meet are called *joints* (Fig. 5). There are *movable* joints, where the bones around the joint move freely, and *immovable* joints, where the bones have fused, like those found in the cranium. A layer of *cartilage*, a very thick and springy tissue, lies over the ends of bones at the joints. Cartilage acts like a rubber padding and absorbs shock.

Around the joint is also found a *capsule* made up of tough fibrous connective tissue. This tissue holds the bones securely together and also permits movement. *Ligaments*, made of the same tough tissue, grow around the entire joint and lash the bones together more securely.

Types of Bones

The following bones make up the human skeleton (Fig. 6):

Long bones are greater in length than in width. They are slightly curved in order to be able to absorb stress. Long bones are found in the legs, toes, arms, forearms, and fingers.

Short bones are cube-shaped, nearly equal in length and width. They are found in the wrists and ankles.

Flat bones are thin and compact bones. They provide protection as well as an area for muscle attachment. The cranium, scapula, ribs, and sternum are examples of flat bones.

Irregular bones are complex-shaped bones that articulate with many other bone surfaces. The vertebra is an irregular bone.

All bones are connected in the body except for the U-shaped hyoid bone found in the throat.

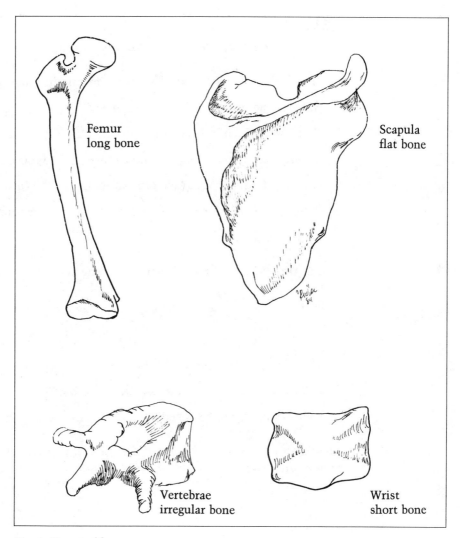

Fig. 6. Types of bones

REVIEW

Indicate whether the following statements are true or false:

1. The skull is an axial bone because it forms the shape of the head and protects the brain. _____ True _____ False

2. Membranes help hold bones together. _____ True _____ False

3. As one grows, many bones tend to fuse. _____ True _____ False

4. The vertebra is an example of a flat bone. _____ True _____ False

5. Upper and lower extremities are made up of appendicular bones. _____ True _____ False

6. List three out of the six functions of the skeletal system.
   a.
   b.
   c.

Fill in the blanks.

7. _____ absorbs shock at the joints.

8. Bones that are cube-shaped are called _____ bones.

Check your answers at the end of the book. If you missed more than one, review the discussion of the skeletal system.

MUSCULAR SYSTEM

Muscles make up the largest mass of tissue in the body and account for 40 to 50 percent of the body's weight. More than 600 muscles assist in moving the skeleton. Muscles provide warmth and strength. Muscles are thick in the middle and taper gradually toward their ends.

There are three different types of muscles that can be identified according to their structure, function, and position.

1. **Smooth muscle**   Found in the walls of the circulatory, digestive, respiratory, reproductive, and excretory organs. Smooth muscle contractions are automatic. Although these muscles respond to nerve impulses, they produce movements that are not usually influenced by the will. Therefore, they are known as *involuntary* muscles. When seen under a microscope, these muscles are not striated (striped).
2. **Cardiac muscle**   Found only in the heart. Like smooth muscle, it is also *involuntary*; however it appears striated. Its special intertwining fibers have the capability of contracting and relaxing the entire heart muscle at rapid intervals.
3. **Voluntary muscle**   For the most part, attached to bones and moves the skeletal system. These are the muscles that can be controlled at will. Voluntary muscle is striated, which makes it thicker, therefore allowing the capability for movement.

Muscle tissue, in combination with various kinds of connective tissue and nerve fibers, make movement possible.

REVIEW

Complete these sentences.

1. Automatic contractions are performed by _____ muscles.

2. Rapid contraction and relaxation is the distinguishing capability of the _____ muscle.

3. Muscle that can be controlled by conscious will is _____ muscle.

4. Muscles provide the body with _____ and _____.

5. Muscles make up approximately _____ of the body's weight.

6. _____ are moved by muscles.

7. Muscles are thick in the middle and _____ toward the end, which enables them to contract and relax.

Check your answers at the end of the book. If you missed any, review the discussion of the muscular system.

MOVEMENT

The point at which two or more bones join together is called a *joint* or *articulation* (Fig. 7). Joints are classified according to their shapes.

1. **Ball and socket**   Joints found in the shoulder and hip that allow the bones to be rotated in a circular manner.
2. **Pivot**   Joints found in the top of the vertebrae of the spine that touch many points of the hinge joint.
3. **Hinge**   Joints found in the knee and elbow.
4. **Condyloid**   Joints found in the wrist and ankle.

Ligaments will sometimes form a capsule around a joint and thereby act as a safety device to prevent injuries.

The joint is considered the center around which the action occurs and is capable of two or more kinds of movement. *Flexion* occurs when the muscle shortens or contracts; one "flexes" the arm or leg. *Extension*, on the other hand, is the straightening or stretching out of the muscle. *Ab-*

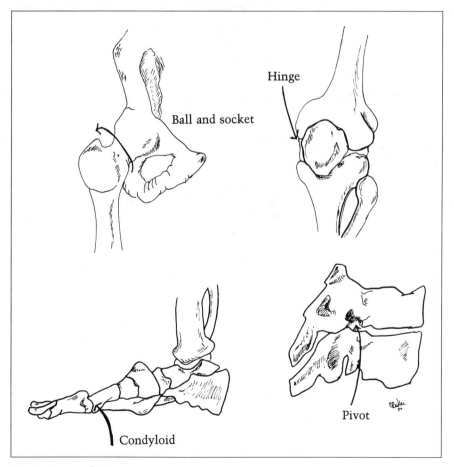

Fig. 7. Types of joints

duction is movement away from the center of the body. *Adduction* is movement toward the center of the body, as when the shoulder is brought down to the side of the body.

The following list of words and Figure 8 deal with movement of the body.

abduct   To move away from the body
adduct   To move toward the body
anterior   Pertaining to the front
distal   Toward the end of a structure
dorsal   Pertaining to the back
inferior   Toward the feet; lower than
lateral   Toward the side of the body
medial   Toward the middle or midline or center of the body
posterior   Pertaining to the back
prone   Lying face down
proximal   Located nearest the center of the body point of attachment to a structure
superior   Toward the head, above another structure
supine   Lying face up
ventral   Pertaining to the front

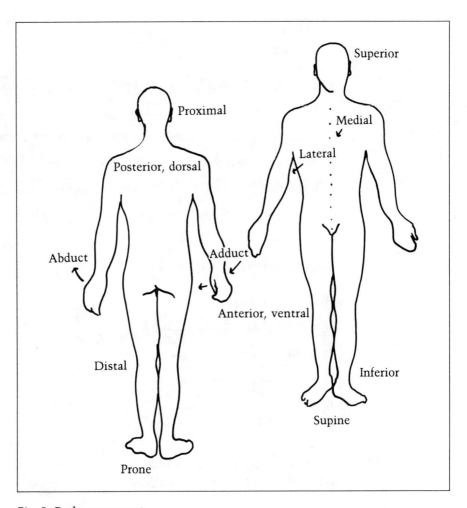

Fig. 8. Body movement

REVIEW

Fill in the correct term.

1. The hip and shoulder are examples of a _____ joint.

2. Joints join two or more _____ together.

3. _____ sometimes cover a joint for protection.

4. When one straightens or stretches a muscle it is called _____

5. Shortening a muscle is called contraction or _____.

6. The point at which two or more bones join together is called _____.

Give the opposite of each term.

7. distal _____

8. medial _____

9. prone _____

10. inferior _____

11. anterior _____

12. adduct _____

Check your answers at the end of the book. If you missed more than one, review the discussion of movement.

Block 1

You are responsible for the following block of terms. Learn Block 1 thoroughly before going on to Block 2. The words are pronounced on the tape. (Practice writing each term five times and think of a word association.)

abdomen	ataxia	cervical	fracture
acetabulum	atrophy	claudication	gluteal
alignment	buttocks	costal	hemiplegia
ambulatory	carpal	emaciated	mediastinum

abdomen (ăb′dō-měn, ăb-dō′měn) Body area between the diaphragm and the pelvis

acetabulum (ăs″ĕ-tăb′ū-lŭm) Socket in the hip bone into which the head of the femur fits (*acid on top of your limb)

alignment (ă-līn′měnt) Formation in a straight line (*the body lined up)

ambulatory (ăm′bū-lăh-tōr″ē) Able to walk (*up to the laboratory)

ataxia (ă-tăks′ĭ-ă) Loss of muscle coordination and power

atrophy (ăt′rō-fē) Wasting away of tissue (*if you do not use your leg muscles in time they will atrophy)

buttocks (bŭt′ŭks) Muscular prominence covering the hip joints

carpal (kar′păl) Pertaining to the wrist

cervical (sĕr′vĭ-kăl) Pertaining to the neck area of the vertebrae

claudication (klaw-dĭ-kā′shŭn) Lameness; limping (*Claudia's vacation)

costal (cŏs′tal) Pertaining to the ribs

emaciated (ē-mā′sĭ-āt-ed) Extremely underweight

fracture (frak′chur) A broken bone

gluteal (gloo′tē-ăl) Of or near the buttocks

hemiplegia (hĕm-ĭ-plē′jĭ-ă) Paralysis of one side of the body

mediastinum (mē″dĭ-ăs-tĭ′nŭm) Middle section of thoracic cavity

REVIEW

Match the following terms with their meanings:

1. costal ____   a. a wasting away of the tissue

2. ataxia ____   b. pertaining to the neck area of vertebra

3. atrophy ____   c. loss of muscle coordination

4. emaciated ____   d. a broken bone

5. fracture ____   e. extremely underweight

6. cervical ____   f. pertaining to the ribs

Fill in the correct term.

7. _____ socket in hip bone into which the head of the femur fits

8. _____ pertaining to the wrist

9. _____ lameness

10. _____ able to walk

Check your answers at the end of the book. If you missed more than one question, review Block 1.

Block 2

Now, go on to Block 2. The terms are pronounced on the tape.

medulla	monoplegia	paraplegia	plantar
membrane	occiput	patella	prosthesis
metacarpus	orthostatic	peripheral	spasmodic
metatarsus	paralysis	phalanges	spastic

medulla (mĕ'-dool'lă)   The inner portion of an organ
membrane (mĕm'brān)   Thin layer or sheet that covers an organ
metacarpus (mĕt"ă-kăr'pŭs)   The part of the hand between wrist and fingers
metatarsus (mĕt"ă-tăr'sŭs)   The part of the foot between the tarsal bones and toes
monoplegia (mŏn-ō-plē'jĭ-ă)   Paralysis of a single (one) limb
occiput (ŏk'sĭ-pŭt)   Back of the head
orthostatic (or"thō-stăt'ĭk)   Pertains to an erect position
paralysis (pă-răl'ĭ-sĭs)   Loss of voluntary motion
paraplegia (păr-ă-plē'jĭ-ă)   Paralysis of the legs
patella (pă-tĕl'ă)   The kneecap
peripheral (pĕr-ĭf'ĕr-ăl)   Pertaining to an outside surface
phalanges (fă-lăn'jēz)   Finger or toe bones
plantar (plăn'tăr)   Pertaining to the sole of the foot
prosthesis (prŏs-thē'sĭs)   Artificial replacement
spasmodic (spăz-mŏd'ĭk)   Sudden tightening, spasmlike
spastic (spăs'tĭk)   Characterized by drawing or stiffening of muscles

Remember, it is not only important to know the meaning of the term but also to pronounce and to spell it correctly!!

REVIEW

Write in the correct term.

patella	membrane	spastic
metacarpus	occiput	plantar
medulla	phalanges	peripheral

1. _____ thin layer that covers organs

2. _____ back of the head

3. _____ pertaining to the sole of the foot

4. _____ inner portion of an organ

5. _____ finger or toe bones

6. _____ kneecap

7. _____ part of the hand between wrist and fingers

Give the meanings of the following terms:

8. prosthesis _____

9. paraplegia _____

10. mediastinum _____

Check your answers at the end of the book. If you missed any, go back and review Section 7. You have been studying the bones of the skeleton.

SEE THE INSTRUCTOR FOR TEST NUMBER 5, WHICH COVERS THE TERMS IN SECTION 7. YOU MUST ACHIEVE AT LEAST 80% MASTERY TO PASS.

It is necessary that you keep reviewing the prefixes, suffixes, and word roots you learned in Sections 1 through 5. This review is to help you continually build on that body of knowledge.

Give the proper definition or medical term for the following:

1. **ostalgia** _____

2. **osteoarthrotomy** _____

3. _____ inflammation of a bone

4. **ostemia** _____

5. **osteoarthritis** _____

6. _____ malignant tumor of brainlike texture in a bone

7. **osteochondritis** _____

8. **osteodystrophia** _____

9. **osteoid** _____

10. _____ softening of a bone

11. **myofibroma** _____

12. _____ muscular tissue cell

13. **myogenesis** _____

14. **myolysis** _____

15. **myoendocarditis** _____

16. _____ rupture of a muscle

17. _____ inflamed condition of muscular tissue of a fallopian tube

18. **arthroscopy** _____

19. _____ disease condition of the joint

20. _____ any joint swelling

21. **arthrodesis** _____

Check your answers at the end of the book. If you had difficulty remembering the terms and meanings, you must review Sections 1 through 4. Another resource besides a medical dictionary is Section 5.

CIRCULATORY AND RESPIRATORY SYSTEMS

CIRCULATORY SYSTEM

The primary functions of the circulatory system are

1. To carry oxygen and nourishment to the body cells
2. To exchange oxygen and nourishment for waste products
3. To carry the waste products to points of elemination

The major organs of the blood circulatory system are

1. Heart
2. Aorta
3. Arteries
4. Arterioles
5. Capillaries
6. Venules and veins
7. Lymph and lymph vessels

As previously discussed, the heart or cardiac muscle, which is the primary organ of the circulatory system, is a striated involuntary muscle that contracts and relaxes about 70 times per minute. This comes to approximately 100,000 heartbeats per day. Each heartbeat pumps about two ounces of blood into the circulatory system, which means about 6,250 quarts of blood are pumped through the heart each day. Generally, the body maintains a steady output of four to six quarts of blood at any given time. Pretty impressive, isn't it!

Blood is made up of a liquid and a solid part. The liquid part consists of plasma, water, chemicals, and dissolved food and salts. The solid part is made up of red corpuscles, white corpuscles, and platelets. Normally the liquid part of the blood has the larger volume of the two parts.

Red corpuscles make up nine-tenths of the cellular amount of blood. There are 250 million red corpuscles in one drop of blood. Red corpuscles contain *hemoglobin* (hemo is the word root for blood), a pigment that carries iron. The hemoglobin combines with oxygen in the lungs, and the red corpuscles carry this oxygen-rich supply to the cells in the body. Red corpuscles live only 50 to 70 days; therefore, they must be continuously replaced. Remember, one of the functions of the skeletal system is to produce red blood cells; this is done in the marrow or inner canal (medulla) of some bones. *Anemia* is a condition that develops when a person lacks iron-rich red blood cells. Red corpuscles have a very definite circular disklike appearance.

White corpuscles have no definite form and move by changing position and shape. White corpuscles destroy bacteria that enter the body; they do this by a method of bacterial engulfment called *phagocytosis*. When bacteria enter the body, the white blood cells are drawn toward the intruder. White cells multiply as they begin to engulf the bacteria. When a "differential" blood study is ordered, the types of white blood cells are examined. A normal total count is 7,500. If the count comes out above this, or if certain types of white blood cells predominate, an inflammation may be suspected. *Leukemia* occurs when there are too many white corpuscles in the body, which rob the body of nutrients and oxygen, thereby depriving normal cells of these vital supplies.

The third cellular component of blood is platelets. Platelets are partially responsible for blood clotting. When there is a break in the skin that disrupts a blood vessel, the blood starts forming pieces of fibrinogen as it flows over the rough broken area. Fibrinogen converts to fibrin, which forms a network to create a dam and stop the blood from escaping from the wound. An excess of platelets can cause clots to form within the system, which in turn can lead to heart attack or stroke. Anticoagulants, that is, medications that interfere with clotting (sometimes called thinners), may be prescribed to patients whose clotting tendency is excessive.

REVIEW

Fill in the blanks.

1. The primary organ of the circulatory system is the _____.

2. The heart is a _____, _____ muscle, which contracts approximately 70 times per minute.

3. State the primary functions of the circulatory system.
   a.
   b.
   c.

4. When there is an extreme lack of iron in the blood, a condition called

   _____ may develop.

5. Bacterial engulfment is called _____.

Check your answers at the end of the book. If you missed any, review the discussion of the circulatory system.

The tubes through which blood flows are called *arteries* and *veins* (Fig. 9); arteries carry blood away from the heart, and veins carry blood toward the heart. The blood circulates through the body by two main pathways (Fig. 10). The first pathway begins at the pulmonary artery. Blood flows from the right side of the heart through the pulmonary artery directly to the lungs to become oxygenated. The pulmonary artery is the only artery in the body that carries nonoxygenated blood. Once the blood is oxygenated, it flows back to the left side of the heart by way of the pulmonary vein (the only vein in the body that carries oxygenated blood).

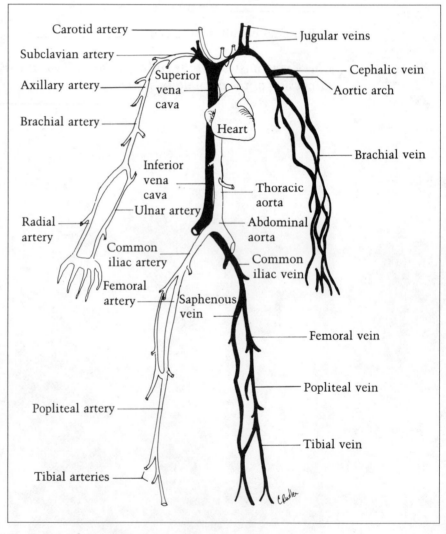

Fig. 9. Vascular system

The second main pathway, beginning at the aorta, carries oxygenated blood away from the left side of the heart to the aortic arch (see Fig. 10) and out to the arteries in the body. From the arteries the blood goes to the arterioles and capillaries, the smallest vascular structures that carry oxygenated blood. From there, the blood starts its climb, by way of the veins, back to the right side of the heart with the waste products it has collected. It travels from the capillaries to the venules, to the veins, and to the vena cava, which enters the heart. Veins have small one-way valves that prevent backflow and assist the blood in its climb back to the heart. Varicose veins develop when these valves break down and collapse, allowing the blood to pool in one spot.

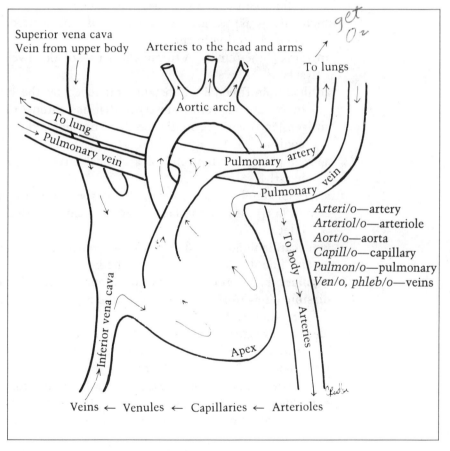

Fig. 10. Circulation through the heart

Block 1

You are responsible for knowing the following medical terms. They are associated with the circulatory system. The words are pronounced on the tape. Try to learn the first block of terms thoroughly before continuing.

anemia	antibody	atrium	diastole
aneurysm	antigen	bradycardia	electrocardiogram
angina	apex	cardiac	embolism
angioma	artery	capillary	embolus

anemia (ăn-ē′mĭ-ă) A deficient number of red blood cells; lack of iron

aneurysm (ăn′ŭ-rĭzm) Weakening of the wall of an artery causing it to balloon out (*'ave you risen?)

angina (ăn-jī′nă) Characterized as a suffocating attack, pain, and an oppressive feeling in the chest

angioma (ăn″jē-ō′mă) A tumor consisting of blood vessels or lymph vessels

antibody (ăn′tī-bŏd″ē) Substance produced by the body to destroy or inactivate a specific substance that has entered the body

antigen (ăn′tĭ-jĕn) A substance that stimulates the production of antibodies

apex (ā′pĕks) Pointed end of a conical structure (pointed end of the heart)

artery (ar′tĕr-ē) Vessel carrying blood away from the heart

atrium (ā′trĭ-ŭm) Chamber or cavity (atrium of each side of the heart) (*let me in)

bradycardia (brād″ĭ-kăr′dĭ-ă) A slow heartbeat (*Brad and Carla)

cardiac (kăr′dē-ăk) Pertaining to the heart

capillary (kăp′ĭ-lăr″ē) Microscopic blood vessel (*Cap or Larry)

diastole (dī-ăs′tō-lē) Relaxation of the heart; bottom number of a blood pressure reading

electrocardiogram (ē-lĕk″trō-kar′dĭ-ŏ-grăm″) Graphic recording of the heart's action potential (abbreviated EKG or ECG)

embolism (ĕm′bō-lĭzm) Obstruction of a blood vessel by foreign matter carried in the blood stream (*an emblem for him)

embolus (ĕm′bō-lŭs) A clot of blood, fat, or air bubble that circulates and lodges in a blood vessel, causing an obstruction

REVIEW

Fill in the correct term.

diastole	**angina**	**artery**
embolus	**antigen**	**capillary**
aneurysm	**apex**	**bradycardia**

1. _____ microscopic blood vessel

2. _____ stimulates production of antibodies

3. _____ pointed end of the conical structure

4. _____ slow heartbeat

5. _____ weakening of the wall of an artery

6. _____ oppressive feeling in the chest

7. _____ clot that causes an obstruction in a blood vessel

Check your answers at the end of the book. If you missed any, review Block 1. After learning these terms completely, continue with Block 2. The terms are pronounced on the tape.

Block 2

hemoglobin	lymphocyte	precordial	valve
hemorrhage	myocardium	pulse	vasospasm
hypertension	occlusion	systole	vein
ischemia	plasma	thrombosis	ventricle
leukocyte			

hemoglobin (hē″mō-glō′bĭn) Iron-containing pigment in the red corpuscles

hemorrhage (hĕm′ĕ-rĭj) Excessive bleeding

hypertension (hĭ″pĕr-tĕn′shŭn) Abnormally high blood pressure

ischemia (ĭs-kē′mĭ-ă) Temporary lack of blood supply to an area (*Is clean a for me a?)

leukocyte (lū′kō-sīt) White blood cell (*Luke's out of sight)

lymphocyte (lĭm′fō-sīt) One type of white blood cell (*limp out of site)

myocardium (mī-ō-kăr′-dĭ-ŭm) Muscle of the heart (*Oh, my car is done!)

occlusion (ō-kloo′zhŭn) The closure of a passage

plasma (plăz′mă) Liquid part of the blood

precordial (prē-kōr′dĭ-ăl) Refers to the region overlying the heart (*he's pretty cordial)

pulse (pŭls) The expansion and contraction of an artery

systole (sĭs′tō-lē) Contraction of the heart muscle; opposite of diastole (*my "sis" told me)

thrombosis (thrŏm-bō′sĭs) Formation of a clot in a blood vessel

valve (vălv) Structure that permits flow of blood in one direction only

vasospasm (vās′ō-spăzm) Constriction of a blood vessel

vein (vān) Vessel carrying blood toward the heart

ventricle (vĕn′trĭk-l) Any small cavity; one of the two chambers of the heart

REVIEW

Match the definition with its correct term.

1. white blood cell ____   a. pulse

2. iron-containing pigment ____   b. occlusion

3. excessive bleeding ____   c. hypertension

4. closure of a passage ____   d. leukocyte

5. liquid part of blood ____   e. hemorrhage

6. expansion and contraction of an artery ____   f. plasma

7. abnormally high blood pressure ____   g. hemoglobin

Check your answers at the end of the book. If you missed any, review Block 2.

Remember, it is important to continually build on the knowledge you gained in the first few sections. Take the following review:

Fill in the correct term or definition as indicated.

   8. **arteriosclerosis** _____

   9. **arteriography** _____

10. _____ artery found below the clavicle

11. **carotid endarterectomy** _____

12. **endarterial** _____

13. **thrombophlebitis** _____

14. _____ inflammation of a vein

15. **aneurysm** _____

16. **myocardial infarction** _____

17. **angiogram** _____

18. _____ inflammation of the heart muscle

19. **cardialgia** _____

20. **cardiomalacia** _____

21. _____ incision of the heart

22. **phleborrhexis** _____

Check your answers at the end of the book. If you are having trouble, go back and review Sections 1 through 4 and consult a medical dictionary for further information.

RESPIRATORY SYSTEM

As discussed previously, the respiratory and circulatory systems work together very closely (Fig. 11). The main organs in the respiratory system are the

1. **Nose** The organ that warms and moistens the incoming air and filters out dirt particles
2. **Pharynx** The passageway for both food and air
3. **Larynx** Located just below the pharynx, it is the beginning of the passageway for air to the lungs; it also aids in voice production
4. **Trachea** The passageway for air to the lungs
5. **Bronchial tubes** Passageways that take the air into the lungs and distribute it into the alveoli (air sacs), where gas exchange occurs
6. **Lungs** Organs in which gas exchange occurs
7. **Diaphragm** The major muscle of respiration

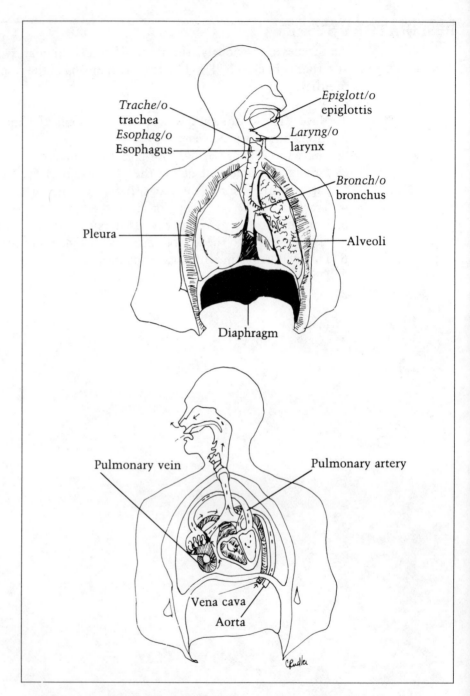

Fig. 11. Respiratory and circulatory systems (dashed lines show flow of oxygen; arrows show flow of carbon dioxide)

Figure 12 illustrates these organs.

The respiratory system provides the following functions:

1. The exchange of gases between the body and its environment
2. The production of sound
3. The elimination of waste gases and water
4. The elimination of excess heat from the body

Respiration occurs through the expansion and recoil of the chest cavity and lungs caused by the action of the diaphragm. The diaphragm is a large muscle that separates the thoracic cavity from the abdominopelvic cavity. During *inhalation*, nerves from the cervical section of the spinal cord stimulate the diaphragm to move downward. This movement causes the ribs to move up and outward, creating a partial vacuum. Air pressure is greater outside the body than in; therefore, when these movements occur, air is forced into the body through the respiratory system. Air is inhaled through the nose or mouth, then pulled down the pharynx,

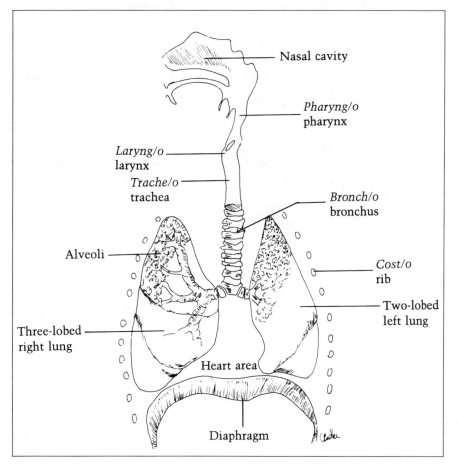

Fig. 12. Respiratory system

larynx, and trachea to the bronchioles and finally into the alveoli. In the alveoli, fresh air is exchanged for waste gases in the blood flowing past.

During *exhalation*, the opposite takes place. The diaphragm relaxes, the ribs move in and down, and the lungs return to their resting state, forcing the air up and out of the body.

All the blood in the body continuously passes through small lung capillaries, which are adjacent to the alveoli (air sacs). The exchange of gases takes place in the alveoli. Venous blood gives up much of the carbon dioxide or waste gases it has picked up from tissue cells in exchange for oxygen present in the alveoli. After this exchange, the blood is oxygenated and its color changes from dark red ("blue" blood) to bright red. Oxygenated blood returns to the heart by way of the pulmonary vein as previously discussed. From the heart, the oxygenated blood is carried through the arteries to tissues throughout the body where oxygen (O_2) is exchanged for carbon dioxide (CO_2) produced in the body cells.

Carbon dioxide is a by-product of *metabolism* and is formed in all tissues. Carbon dioxide crosses the cell membrane and enters the bloodstream as the blood gives up its oxygen supply to the cell. The carbon dioxide is then carried by the circulatory system back to the lungs where it crosses the membrane of the alveoli in exchange for oxygen, and the cycle begins again.

As one can see, the respiratory system is closely linked to the circulatory system as well as to the nervous system, the latter providing the stimulus that causes the diaphragm to contract.

Block 1

The following medical terms are associated with the respiratory system. You are responsible for knowing them. They are pronounced on your tape. Learn them thoroughly before going on to Block 2.

anoxia	**bronchus**	**dyspnea**	**exhalation**
apnea	**cyanosis**	**emphysema**	**hemoptysis**
asphyxia	**diaphragm**	**eupnea**	**hypoxia**

anoxia (ăn-ŏks′ĭ-ă)   Deficient oxygen (O_2) supply to the tissues

apnea (ăp′nē-ă)   Temporary cessation of breathing

asphyxia (ăs-fĭk′sĭ-ă)   Suffocation; condition characterized by anoxia

bronchus (brŏng′kŭs)   One of the two branches of the trachea

cyanosis (sī-ăn-ō′sĭs)   Bluish appearance of the skin due to reduced oxygen supply in the blood

diaphragm (dī′ă-frăm)   Muscular partition between the thorax and abdomen

dyspnea (dĭsp′nē-ă)   The sensation of difficult or labored breathing

emphysema (ĕm″fĭ-sē′mă)   Disease characterized by dilatation of pulmonary alveoli

eupnea (ŭp′nē-ă)   Normal respiration
exhalation (ĕks″hă-lā′shŭn)   Process of breathing out
hemoptysis (hē-mŏp′tĭ-sĭs)   Coughing up of blood
hypoxia (hī″pŏks′ĭ-ă)   Lack of adequate amount of oxygen in inhaled air

Block 2

hypoxemia	**inhalation**	**orthopnea**
hypercapnia	**metabolism**	**respiration**
hyperventilation	**naris**	**pulmonary**

hypoxemia (hī-pŏks-ē′mĭ-ă)   Insufficient oxygenation of the blood
hypercapnia (hī-pĕr-kăp′nĭ-ă)   Large amount of carbon dioxide in the blood
hyperventilation (hī′pĕr-vĕn-tĭ-lā′shŭn)   Increased inhalation and exhalation as a result of an increase in rate or depth of respiraton or both
inhalation (ĭn″hă-lā′shŭn)   The act of drawing in breath
metabolism (mĕ-tăb′ō-lĭzm)   Process by which food is used by a living organism
naris (nă′rĭs)   Nostril
orthopnea (or″thŏp′nē-ă)   Inability to breathe while lying down
respiration (rĕs″pĭr-ā′shŭn)   The act of breathing
pulmonary (pŭl′mō-nă-rē)   Involving the lungs

Write every word five times to help you remember them.

REVIEW

Match the following terms to their meanings:

1. naris _____
2. apnea _____
3. hyperventilation _____
4. metabolism _____
5. hypercapnia _____
6. asphyxia _____
7. emphysema _____
8. dyspnea _____
9. cyanosis _____
10. anoxia _____

a. suffocation
b. increased inhalation and exhalation
c. disease of pulmonary alveoli
d. nostril
e. deficient oxygen supply to tissues
f. sensation of difficult breathing
g. bluish skin appearance
h. temporary cessation of breathing
i. large amount of carbon dioxide in blood
j. process by which food is used by an organism

Check your answers at the end of the book. If you missed any, go back and restudy Blocks 1 and 2.

Fill in the proper term or definition pertaining to the respiratory system.

1. **rhinitis** _____

2. _____ removal of a lung

3. **bronchiectasis** _____

4. _____ originating in the bronchus

5. **thoracentesis** _____

6. **bronchogram** _____

7. _____ inflammation of the lung

8. _____ incision made into the trachea

9. _____ visualization of esophagus with a scope

10. **tracheomalacia** _____

Check your answers at the end of the book. If you missed any, review Blocks 1 and 2 and the prefixes, suffixes, and word roots.

Continue your review with the Anatomy and Physiology Mid-Review *before taking Test Number 6.*

ANATOMY AND PHYSIOLOGY MID-REVIEW

This review covers Sections 6, 7, and 8.

1. State the four major body cavities.
   a.
   b.
   c.
   d.

2. The smallest structural unit of all things is the _____.

3. State three purposes of the skeletal system.
   a.
   b.
   c.

4. An immovable joint can be found in the _____.

5. Axial bones protect and form. What is an example of an axial bone?

   _____

6. State three types of bones.
   a.
   b.
   c.

7. Smooth muscles, found in such areas as the digestive and respiratory systems, are also called _____ muscles.

8. The heart is a _____, _____ muscle.

9. A person with an iron deficiency is said to be _____.

10. An _____ is a vessel that carries blood away from the heart.

11. The knee is an example of a _____ joint.

12. _____ is movement of a limb toward the center of the body.

13. A person who has an unusually slow heartbeat has _____.

14. The region lying over the area of the heart is the _____ area.

15. The phase of breathing in which air is taken into the lungs is

    _____.

16. The phase of breathing in which air is expelled from the lungs is

    _____.

17. The muscle that moves downward in the inhalation phase of breathing is the _____.

18. Lack of oxygen in the tissue is called _____.

Circle the correct spelling and give the definitions of the following terms:

1. ETEOLOGY   ETIOLOGY   ETTEOLOGY

_____

2. SYNDROME   SYMDROME   SINDROME

_____

3. ACETABULUM   ACITABULUM   ACIDTABULUM

_____

4. LION   LOYN   LOIN

_____

5. PERIFERAL   PERIPHERAL   PERIPHEREL

_____

6. DEASTOLE   DIASTOLE   DIASTOLIE

_____

7. ANEURYSM   ANURYSM   ANEURISM

_____

8. ISKEMIA   ISHKEMIA   ISCHEMIA

_____

9. HEMOPTASIS   HEMOPTYSIS   HEMAPTOSIS

_____

10. ORTHOPNEA   ORTHOPNIA   ORTOPNEA

_____

Match each term with its proper meaning:

1. eupnea _____   a. word root meaning breathing

2. dyspnea _____   b. normal breathing

3. hyperpnea _____   c. sensation of difficult breathing

4. orthopnea _____   d. breathing too rapidly

5. apnea _____   e. breathing too deeply

6. tachypnea _____   f. temporary cessation of breathing

7. pnea _____   g. inability to breathe while lying down

Unscramble the following terms:

1. formation of a clot in a blood vessel
   (bmhrossiot)   _____
2. white blood cell
   (coklteeuy)   _____
3. constriction of a blood vessel
   (oapassmvs)   _____
4. abnormally high blood pressure
   (yetninhpreso)   _____
5. involving the lung
   (umnryploa)   _____

Check your answers at the end of the book. If you missed more than two, review Sections 6 through 8.

SEE THE INSTRUCTOR FOR TEST NUMBER 6, WHICH COVERS THE CIRCULATORY AND RESPIRATORY SYSTEMS. YOU MUST ACHIEVE AT LEAST 80% MASTERY TO PASS.

URINARY SYSTEM

The urinary system removes wastes from the blood and eliminates them from the body. The study of this system is called *urology*.

The urinary system (also called the *excretory system*) is made up of a pair of *kidneys*, which are located at the lower part of the back above the hips. They are well padded by a layer of fat. The basic functions of the kidneys are to

1. Filter dissolved substances (amino acids, ammonia, urea, and sugar) and water from the blood
2. Reabsorb those filtered substances and water back into the blood minus waste materials
3. Secrete waste materials out from the body in the form of urine

The two *ureters* carry the urine from the kidneys to the *bladder*. The bladder is made up of involuntary muscles and can stretch to a large size. Urine is stored in the bladder until there is a large enough quantity for the body to feel the urge to *void*, or urinate. The *urethra* is the passageway through which urine is discarded to the outside of the body (Fig. 13).

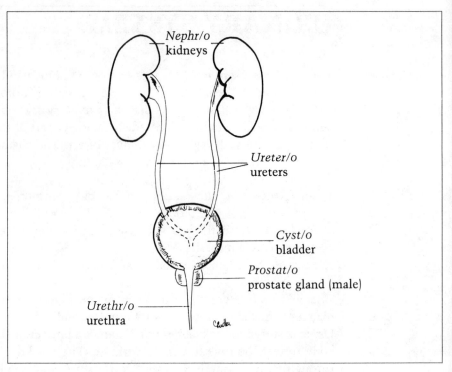

Fig. 13. Urinary system

Block 1

The following medical terms are associated with the urinary system. You are responsible for knowing them. The words are pronounced on your tape. Learn them thoroughly before going on to the next section.

bladder	elimination	hematuria	polyuria
catheter	enuresis	incontinent	pyuria
cortex	glucose	micturition	renal
dysuria	glycosuria	oliguria	void
edema			

bladder (blă'dĕr)   A sac collecting fluid
catheter (kăth'ĕt-ĕr)   A tube for evacuating or injecting fluids through a natural passage; made of plastic, rubber, glass, or metal
cortex (kŏr'tĕks)   Outer part of an internal organ; cortex of the kidney
dysuria (dĭs-ū'rĭ-ă)   Difficult or painful urination
edema (ĕ-dē'mă)   Swelling from excessive fluid in a tissue
╋ **elimination** (ē-lĭm'ĭ-nā-shŭn)   Expulsion of wastes from the body
enuresis (ĕn"ū-rē'sĭs)   Involuntary urination (bed-wetting)
glucose (gloo'kōs)   Form of sugar that normally is entirely reabsorbed by the blood
╋ **glycosuria** (glī"kō-soo'rĭ-ă)   Sugar in the urine
hematuria (hē"mă-tū'rĭ-ă)   Blood in the urine
incontinent (ĭn-con'tĭ-nĕnt)   Inability to control the elimination of urine or feces
micturition (mĭk-tū-rĭ'shŭn)   The act of urinating
oliguria (ŏl-ĭg-ū'rĭ-ă)   Decreased production of urine
polyuria (pŏl"ē-ū'rĭ-ă)   Excessive discharge of urine
pyuria (pĭ-ū'rĭ-ă)   Pus in the urine
renal (rē'năl)   Pertaining to the kidneys
void (voyd)   To cast out as waste matter; to urinate

REVIEW

Supply the word that completes these sentences.

1. The urinary system is also called the _excretory_ system.
2. The _kidneys_ filter waste materials from the blood and produce urine.
3. The _ureters_ carry urine from the kidneys into the bladder.
4. The _bladder_ is a sac that holds urine until a sufficient amount is collected.
5. The _urethra_ is the passageway through which urine leaves the body.

Match the following terms with their proper meanings:

6. incontinent _f_   a. sugar in the urine
7. dysuria _d_   b. involuntary urination (bed-wetting)
8. pyuria _c_   c. pus in the urine
9. hematuria _g_   d. difficult or painful urination
10. enuresis _b_   e. decreased production of urine
11. glycosuria _a_   f. inability to control elimination
12. oliguria _e_   g. blood in the urine

Check your answers at the end of the book. If you missed more than one, review this section.

Complete the following with the correct term or definition:

13. _____ inflammation of the bladder

14. **ureterolithotomy** _____

15. _____ inflammation of the kidney pelvis

16. **ureterostomy** _____

17. **nephrocele** _____

18. **nephropexy** _____

19. _____ droopy bladder

Check your answers at the end of the book. Try to keep up with a continuous review of prefixes, suffixes, and word roots.

Now, go on to Section 10, Digestive System.

DIGESTIVE SYSTEM

Nourishment is required for survival. The digestive system is responsible for making the nourishment taken in during eating available to body cells, where it can be either stored or used for energy. This system also eliminates from the body the wastes resulting from the digestive process.

Food must undergo many changes from the time it enters the body through the mouth to the time it is ready to be used for nourishment. The digestive system has two important functions:

1. To convert food to a state capable of being absorbed by the cells. This process is both mechanical and chemical. Mechanically, the food is moved along the tract and broken into fine particles (*mastication*). Chemically, the stomach, gallbladder, liver, and pancreas produce enzymes that attack the food and break it into still smaller pieces. The chemical process prepares the way for the second phase of the digestive process.
2. To transfer the digested food from the intestinal tract into the bloodstream, which is *absorption*. Remember, it is the circulatory system that carries the nutrients to the body's cells.

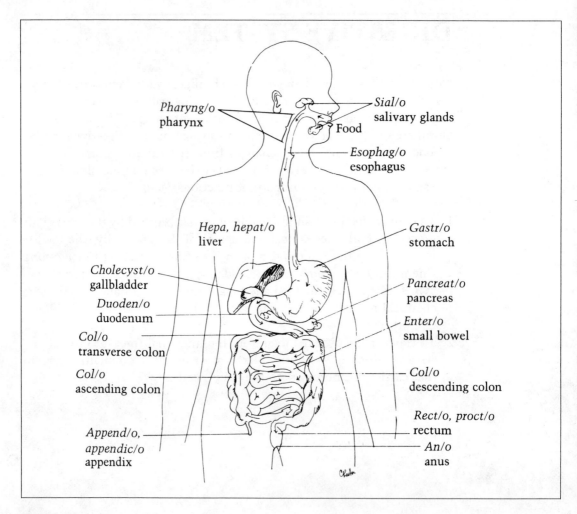

Fig. 14. Digestive system

If one were to follow the food as it passes through the digestive system (Fig. 14), one would travel:

1. From the *mouth*
2. To the *pharynx*
3. Into the *esophagus*
4. Down to the *stomach*
5. Into the *small bowel*
6. Into the *colon*
7. Into the *rectum* to the *anus*, where the waste material is expelled

The total passageway has several names: the *digestive tract*, the *gastro-intestinal tract*, and the *alimentary canal*. *Gastroenterology* is the study of the digestive system.

The organs of this system ingest, chew, swallow, and push food down into the stomach. Here gastric juices produced by *glands* in the stomach wall convert solid particles of food to a semiliquid state. The stomach releases small amounts of this semiliquid into the small bowel (or intestine). The small bowel is a tube approximately 1 to 1½ inches in circumference and approximately 23 feet long. It is convoluted (folded) so it can fit compactly into the abdominal cavity. In the small bowel, other digestive juices that contribute to the chemical process of food breakdown are released from accessory organs. The accessory organs are the *pancreas*, *liver*, and *gallbladder*. The digestive juices produced by these organs help further break down the semiliquid. The nutrients from the ingested food begin to be absorbed into tiny capillaries and lymph vessels in the walls of the small bowel. Ingested food remaining in the small bowel after absorption has taken place moves on into the colon. Here, water is reabsorbed into the bloodstream leaving a semisolid residual within the bowel. Finally, semisolid waste products (what is left over) are eliminated from the body through the anus (mechanical process).

REVIEW

1. What are some other names for the digestive system?
   a.
   b.

2. What are the two functions of the digestive system?
   a.
   b.

3. As the food travels through the system, what is it that aids in the chemical breakdown?

Check your answers at the end of the book. If you missed any, review the discussion on the digestive system.

Block 1

The following medical terms are associated with the digestive system. You are responsible for knowing them. The terms are pronounced on the tape. Try to learn the first block thoroughly before continuing.

anastomosis	calculus	crepitus	edentia
anorexia	caries	defecation	emesis
anus	cholecystitis	dehydration	enteritis
appendectomy	colic	dysphagia	eructation
cachexia	colon		

anastomosis (ă-năs"tō-mō'sĭs)   Connection between hollow tubes; most frequently used in surgery to connect two parts of the bowel after a resection

anorexia (ăn-ō-rĕks'ĭ-ă)   Loss of appetite¹

anus (ā'nŭs)   Outlet of the rectum

appendectomy (ăp"ĕn-dĕk'tō-mē)   Removal of the appendix

cachexia (kă-kĕks'ĭ-ă)   Ill health from malnutrition

calculus (kăl'kū-lŭs)   Stone formed in the body

caries (kār'ēz)   Decay of tooth or bone

✗ **cholecystitis** (kō"lē-sĭs-tī'tĭs)   Inflammation of the gallbladder

colic (kŏl'ĭk)   Severe spasmodic intestinal pain

colon (kō'lŏn)   Large intestine

crepitus (krĕp'ĭ-tŭs)   Noise of gas discharged from the intestine; crackling sound

defecation (dĕf-ĕ-kā'shŭn)   Elimination of waste from the rectum

dehydration (dē"hī-drā'shŭn)   A condition resulting from extreme loss of water from tissue

dysphagia (dĭs-fā'jĭ-ă)   Inability to swallow as a result of spasm of the esophagus

edentia (ē-dĕn'shĭ-ă)   The condition of being without teeth; refers to a diet ordered for someone without teeth

emesis (ĕm'ĕs-ĭs)   Vomiting

enteritis (ĕn"tĕr-ī'tĭs)   Inflammation of the intestines

eructation (ē-rŭk-tā'shŭn)   Belching

REVIEW

Fill in the proper term.

defecation	**anorexia**	**dehydration**
anus	**emesis**	**cachexia**
edentia	**colic**	**caries**

1. decay of teeth or bones _____

2. ill health from malnutrition _____

3. elimination of wastes from the rectum _____

4. a condition resulting from extreme loss of water from tissue

   _____

5. loss of appetite _____

6. vomiting _____

7. condition of being without teeth _____

8. severe spasmodic intestinal pain _____

Check your answers at the end of the book. If you missed any, review Block 1.

Block 2

Continue with Block 2. Play the tape; the words are pronounced for you. Try writing each term five times to help you remember how to spell it.

flatus	**hematemesis**	**mastication**	**peristalsis**
gastric	**hernia**	**obese**	**rectum**
gavage	**jaundice**	**palate**	**singultus**
gingivitis	**lipid**	**parorexia**	**uvula**
glossal			

flatus (flā′tŭs)   Expulsion of air (gas) from the bowel

gastric (găs′trĭc)   Pertaining to the stomach

gavage (gă-vazh′)   Nourishment given through a tube into the stomach

gingivitis (jĭn-jĭ-vī′tĭs)   Inflammation of the gums

glossal (glŏs′săl)   Pertaining to the tongue

hematemesis (hĕm-ăt-ĕm′ē-sĭs)   Blood in vomitus

hernia (hĕr′nĭ-ă)   Protrusion of part of an organ through the wall that normally contains it

jaundice (jawn′dĭs)   Yellow discoloration of skin

lipid (lĭp′-ĭd)   Fatlike tissue

mastication (măs-tĭ-kā′shŭn)   Chewing

obese (ō-bēs′)   Extremely fat

palate (păl′ăt)   The roof of the mouth

parorexia (păr-ō-rĕk′sĭ-ă)   An abnormal craving for food

peristalsis (pĕr-ĭ-stăl′sĭs)   A wavelike movement in the digestive organs that propels the contents forward

rectum (rĕk′tŭm)   Last five inches of the colon

singultus (sĭng-gŭl′tŭs)   Hiccups

uvula (ū′vū-lă)   Small soft structure hanging from free edge of the roof of the mouth

REVIEW

Circle the correct spellings and give the definitions.

1. GLOSSEL   GLOSSAL   GLOSAL

_____

2. JAUNDICE   JOHNDICE   JONDICE

_____

3. HEMATAMESIS   HEMATEMESIS   HEMOTAMESIS

_____

4. SINGUTIS   SINGILTUS   SINGULTUS

_____

5. PERISTALSIS   PERASTALSIS   PARASTALSIS

_____

Fill in the correct terms.

6. inflammation of the gums _____

7. expulsion of air (gas) from the bowel _____

8. abnormal craving for food _____

9. extremely fat _____

10. roof of mouth _____

Check your answers at the end of the book. If you missed any, review Block 2.

Fill in the proper terms or definitions for the following:

11. _____ removal of part or all of the stomach

12. _____ making a more or less permanent opening into
    the colon

13. **enteritis** _____

14. **choledochotomy** _____

15. **enterocele** _____

16. _____ a tube put into the stomach

17. **esophagospasm** _____

18. _____ visualization of the esophagus

19. **hepatomegaly** _____

20. _____ upper stomach hernia

21. _____ formation of stones in the gallbladder

22. **stomatoma** _____

23. **proctoscopy** _____

Check your answers at the end of the book. If you missed any, be sure to review Section 5.

REPRODUCTIVE SYSTEM

FEMALE

There are three functions of the female reproductive system.

1. Renewal of life
2. Secretion of hormones to stimulate body development and feminine characteristics, help regulate the menstrual cycle, and make pregnancy possible
3. Sexual gratification

The reproductive organs of the female include

1. The uterus
2. Two fallopian tubes
3. Two ovaries
4. The vagina

The breasts, or mammary glands, are also considered part of the reproductive system (Fig. 15A).

Before the female child enters her tenth or eleventh year of life, her reproductive organs grow slowly. Around the age of twelve, hormone production begins to stimulate the body to transform gradually toward womanhood. Hair growth appears, breasts grow, and menstruation begins. This period of time is termed *puberty*. The female is now capable of becoming pregnant.

Menstruation

Each month, one of the two ovaries produces an egg (ovum). This is termed *ovulation*. The egg is released from the ovary and travels into the fallopian tube. It slowly passes from the fallopian tube into the uterus. If during the egg's journey through the fallopian tube it is penetrated by a male's sperm, the egg becomes fertile. The fertile egg then travels into the uterus and implants itself in the uterine wall. Here it grows into a baby. If the egg is not fertilized, it passes through the uterus and out of the body in a bloody discharge called *menses*. The bloody discharge comes from the lining of the uterus, which has been preparing to nourish a fertile egg all month. When an egg does not become fertile, the lining is shed. After about five days, the bleeding ceases and the cycle begins again.

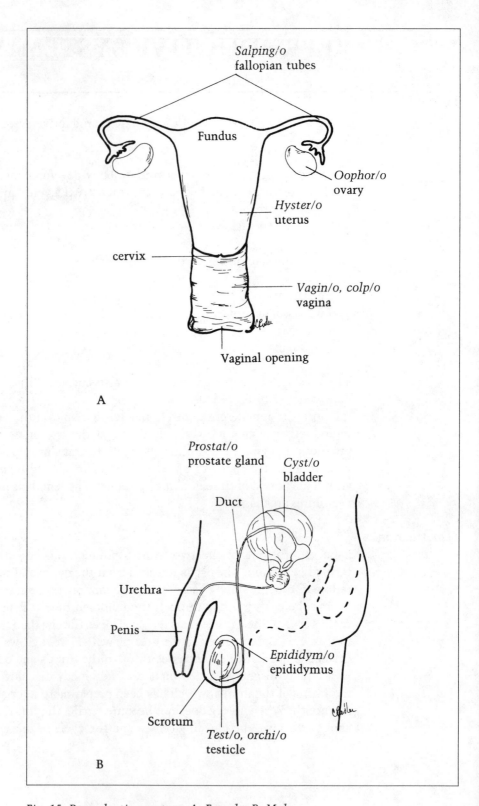

Fig. 15. Reproductive system. A. Female. B. Male

MALE

The primary functions of the male reproductive system are

1. Reproduction
2. Hormonal secretion
3. Sexual gratification

The reproductive organs are

1. A pair of male sex glands (testes)
2. A series of internal ducts (tubular vessels that carry gland secretions)
3. The scrotum
4. The penis

These organs are illustrated in Figure 15B.

Before the early teens, both the male and female reproductive systems develop slowly. In the male, puberty is marked by physical changes: growth of hair, deepening of voice, and increase of muscle mass. From the age of puberty, the internal duct system is continually secreting spermatozoa, which have the capability of fertilizing the female's egg. In the scrotum and penis, there is a special kind of tissue called *erectile tissue*. When stimulated, this tissue becomes engorged with blood and causes the organ to become large and rigid, enabling it to be introduced into the female vagina and deposit sperm there.

Block 1

The following medical terms are associated with the reproductive system. You are responsible for knowing them. They are pronounced on your tape. Try to learn them completely before continuing.

adolescence	embryo	lactation	puberty
amenorrhea	fetus	mammary	primipara
dysmenorrhea	fundus	multipara	umbilicus
ectopic pregnancy	gestation	postpartum	

adolescence (ăd″ō-lĕs′ĕns)   The period from the beginning of puberty until adulthood

amenorrhea (ā-mĕn″ō-rē′ă)   Absence or supression of menstrual flow

dysmenorrhea (dĭs″mĕn-ō-rē′ă)   Painful or difficult menstruation

ectopic pregnancy (ĕk-tŏp′ĭk)   Implantation of the fertilized egg cell outside of the uterus, frequently, the fallopian tube

embryo (ĕm′brĭ-ō)   The developing human from the second week in utero to the eighth week

fetus (fē′tŭs)   The developing human from the third month in utero to birth

fundus (fŭn′dŭs)   The larger part of a hollow organ (uterus)

gestation (jĕs-tā′shŭn)   Period of intrauterine fetal development; in a human, nine months

lactation (lăk-tā′shŭn)   The period of suckling a child

mammary (măm′ă-rē)   Pertaining to the breast

multipara (mŭl-tĭp′ă-ră)   A woman who has borne more than one child

postpartum (pōst-păr′tŭm)   The period after delivery of newborn (adjective form)

puberty (pū′bĕr-tē)   Period in life when sex organs become active and are capable of reproduction

primipara (prē-mĭp′ă-ră)   A woman who has given birth to her first child

umbilicus (ŭm-bĭl′ĭ′kŭs)   The navel; former attachment of mother to fetus

REVIEW

Match the following terms to their definitions:

1. ectopic pregnancy _e_   a. a developing human between second and eighth week in utero

2. fetus _c_   b. absence of menstruation

3. amenorrhea _b_   c. a developing human between third month in utero and birth

4. gestation _f_   d. puberty until adulthood

5. primipara _g_   e. implantation of a fertilized egg outside of the uterus

6. adolescence _d_   f. period of intrauterine development

7. embryo _a_   g. woman who has given birth to her first child

Check your answers at the end of the book. If you missed any, go back and review Block 1.

Fill in the proper terms or definitions.

8. _____ removal of the uterus

9. _____ drooping testicles

10. _____ plastic repair of the uterus

11. _____ removal of part or entire vas deferens

12. **oophoralgia** _____

13. **hysteropexy** _____

14. _____ removal of right fallopian tube and ovary

Check your answers at the end of the book. Review Section 5 if you missed any.

SEE THE INSTRUCTOR TO TAKE TEST NUMBER 7, WHICH WILL COVER SECTIONS 9, 10, AND 11. YOU MUST ACHIEVE AT LEAST 80% MASTERY TO PASS.

ENDOCRINE AND NERVOUS SYSTEMS

ENDOCRINE SYSTEM

The endocrine system is made up of a group of glands that greatly influence growth and development (Fig. 16). *Endocrine* means to secrete internally. Endocrine glands produce special chemicals called *hormones* that are secreted into the circulatory system and carried to specific organs where they exert certain regulatory functions. The major glands of the endocrine system are as follows:

1. **Pituitary** Composed of two glands, one anterior and one posterior. Mushroom-shaped, it lies deep within the cranial cavity attached to the base of the brain (hypothalamus). The pituitary is often referred to as the "master gland," because four of the six anterior pituitary hormones act on other endocrine glands to regulate their activity. The remaining two hormones of the anterior pituitary and the two hormones from the posterior pituitary directly regulate the following:

   1. Growth, development, and sexual maturation
   2. Water balance in the blood and tissues
   3. Chemical balance in blood and tissue fluids
   4. Physiologic muscle movement to begin and maintain labor
   5. Lactation in the female

2. **Thyroid** Found in the neck area below the larynx, its hormones help regulate normal growth and development and body metabolism. This gland stores iodine (a chemical element) and regulates its secretion into the bloodstream. Iodine regulates the amount of energy cells release to get their work done.
3. **Parathyroid** Found at the back of the thyroid, the four small parathyroid glands help maintain normal calcium and phosphorus levels in the blood.
4. **Adrenal** There are two adrenals, one located superior to each kidney. Each adrenal is really two glands in one; the adrenal *cortex* produces three hormones that influence chemical electrolyte balance, metabolism, and sexual characteristics. The adrenal *medulla* produces two hormones that help the body react to stress.
5. **Thymus** Found in the neck behind the sternum between the lungs. It does not secrete any known hormone; however, scientists believe it is instrumental in the development of the body's immune system.

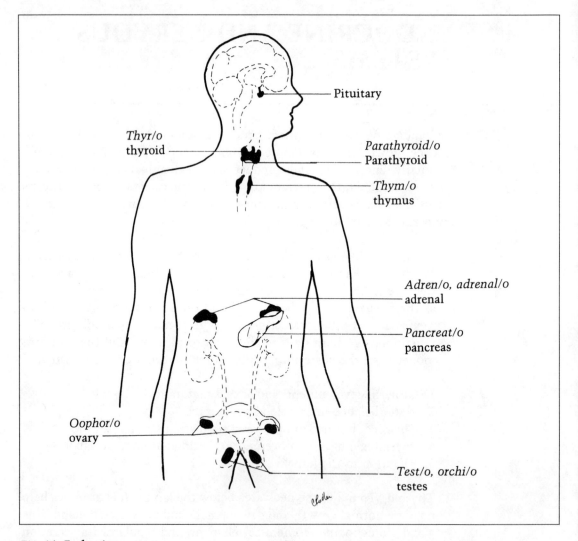

Fig. 16. Endocrine system

6. **Endocrine pancreas (islets of Langerhans)** Found posterior to the stomach, the pancreas is firmly attached to the duodenum and stretches to the spleen. It produces two hormones that regulate the body's blood sugar level.
7. **Ovaries** Found only in the female, the ovaries produce hormones that influence female characteristics, menses, and pregnancy.
8. **Testes** Found only in the male, the testes secrete a hormone that influences male characteristics.

NERVOUS SYSTEM

The *central nervous system (CNS)* is made up of the brain and spinal cord (Fig. 17). The *peripheral nervous system* is made up of all the body's nerves. All body systems are dependent on the nervous system. This system controls

1. Consciousness
2. Mental processes
3. Regulation of body movements and functions through the dispatch of nerve impulses involving all areas of the body

Nature provides a measure of protection to the brain and the spinal cord since their functions are essential to life. Thus the brain is encased inside the skull, and the spinal cord is enclosed within a canal that goes down the center of the bony vertebral column.

Central Nervous System

The brain is divided into seven parts.

1. **Cerebrum**   The center for mental processes of all types: sensations, consciousness, and control of voluntary movements. The cerebrum is the largest section of the brain.
2. **Cerebellum**   The center for muscular coordination and balance. The cerebellum is the second largest area of the brain.
3. **Hypothalamus**   Controls hormonal secretion through the pituitary gland, the functioning of most internal organs, appetite, and reward and punishment centers.
4. **Thalamus**   Located within each half, or hemisphere, of the cerebrum, it controls sensations and emotions.
5. **Medulla, pons, and midbrain**   Collectively referred to as the *brain stem*, these structures form the lowest part of the brain and also the enlarged part of the spinal cord within the cranial cavity. This vital section controls blood pressure, respiration, heartbeat, and the diameter of blood vessels.

The spinal cord is the center for all spinal cord reflexes. The sensory tracts send impulses to the brain, and motor tracts send impulses from the brain.

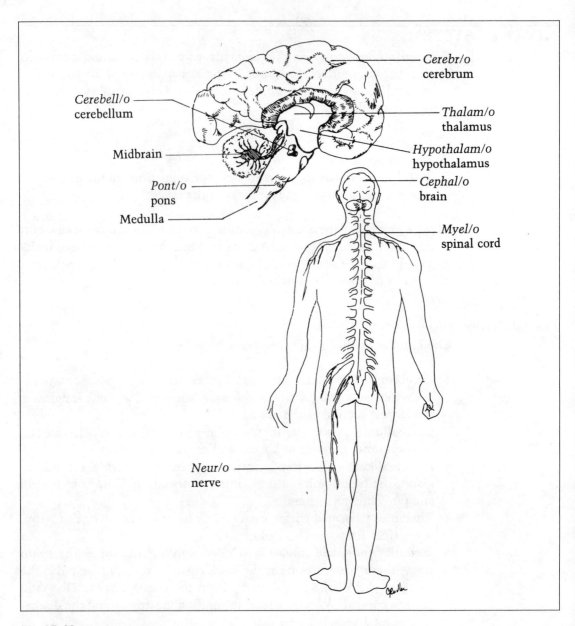

Fig. 17. Nervous system

Peripheral Nervous System

The peripheral nervous system (PNS) includes all nerves that extend from the CNS to all parts of the body. Within the PNS there are basic types of nerves that control specific functions and reactions.

1. **Cranial nerves** Twelve pairs of nerves that send impulses between the brain and structures in the head, the neck, and the thoracic and abdominal cavities (e.g., certain pairs control hearing, while others control shoulder and head movements).
2. **Spinal nerves** Thirty-one pairs of nerves attached to the spinal cord that send and receive impulses between the spinal cord and all areas not supplied with cranial nerves. Spinal nerves control both sensation and movement. Therefore, if the spinal cord is damaged, feeling or movement may be absent below the damaged area.
3. **Autonomic nerves** A group of nerves that cannot be controlled voluntarily. For example, a person can control eye movements but not the amount the body perspires. There are **sympathetic** and **parasympathetic** autonomic nerve fibers. Under normal unstressful situations, the parasympathetic fibers of the autonomic nerve dominate. For example, these nerves keep heartbeat, blood pressure, and perspiration normal. Under mental or physical tension, sympathetic fibers dominate and create certain rapid changes within the body: when frightened, "goose pimples" appear, pupils dilate, and the heart beats more rapidly.

Again, we have just scratched the surface of these complicated systems, and there is much more involved than what has been discussed here. There are, however, a few medical terms for the most part associated with the nervous system that you are responsible for knowing. They are pronounced on the tape for you. Try to learn them thoroughly before going on.

Block 1

aphasia	hallucination	paroxysm
cephalalgia	hydrocephalus	psychosomatic
coma	incoherence	syncope
electroencephalogram	lethargy	vertigo

aphasia (ă-fā′zĭ-ă)   A loss of ability to speak, write, or comprehend

cephalalgia (sĕf-ă-lăl′jĭ-ă)   Headache

coma (cō′mă)   Unconsciousness with complete lack of response to stimuli

electroencephalogram (ē-lĕk″trō-ĕn-sĕf′ă-lō-grăm)   Graphic record of the brain's electrical activity (abbreviated EEG)

hallucination (hă-loo-sĭ-na′shun)   A perception (visual or auditory) not based on reality

hydrocephalus (hī-drō-sĕf′ă-lŭs)   Abnormal increase in cerebrospinal fluid around the brain

incoherence (in″kō-hēr′ĕns)   Inability to express oneself rationally

lethargy (lĕth-ăr′gē)   Mental dullness or drowsiness

paroxysm (păr′ŏk-sĭzm)   Convulsion

psychosomatic (sī″kō-sō-măt′ĭk)   Referring to the influence of the mind, primarily emotions, on the body's physical functions

syncope (sĭn′kŭ-pē)   Fainting

vertigo (vĕr′tĭ-gō)   A sensation of dizziness

REVIEW

Fill in the terms that best complete these sentences.

1. The technical term for a headache is _cephalalgia_

2. The development of excess cerebrospinal fluid around the brain is called _hydrocephalus_

3. When one's physical symptoms are influenced by an emotional state, the symptoms are said to be _psychosomatic_

4. The state of being unable to express oneself rationally is called _incoherence_

5. The sensation of dizziness is called _vertigo_.

6. Endocrine glands produce _hormones_

7. The _pituitary_ gland is referred to as the "master gland" because it regulates the activity of the other glands in the endocrine system.

8. The spinal cord's natural protection is the _vert. column_

Complete the following with the correct terms:

9. The functions of the peripheral nervous system are to:
   a. _consciousness_
   b. _body movements_   _mental processes_

10. The three basic types of nerves that make up the peripheral nervous system are:
    a. _autonomic_
    b. _cranial_
    c. _spinal_

11. Your _____ _a._ _____ react when you are in an anxious state.
    a. sympathetic fibers
    b. parasympathetic fibers

Check your answers at the end of the book. Review Block 1 if you missed any.

MORE MEDICAL TERMS

In this section, common medical terms are introduced for learning. They are presented in blocks and pronounced on the tape. Please learn one block completely before continuing to the next block.

Block 1

abnormal	**afebrile**	**asepsis**	**biopsy**
abscess	**alkalosis**	**aspirate**	**cataract**
acidosis	**amblyopia**	**axilla**	**cerumen**
acute	**ascites**	**autopsy**	**cholesterol**

abnormal (ăb-nōr′măl)   That which is not normal

abscess (ăb′sĕs)   Localized collection of pus in a cavity or tissue

acidosis (ăs″ĭ-dō′sĭs)   Condition in which there is an excessive amount of acid in the blood

acute (ă-cūt′)   Sharp, severe

afebrile (ă-fĕb′rĭl)   Without fever

alkalosis (ăl-kă-lō′sĭs)   Condition in which there is too much alkali in the blood

amblyopia (ăm″blĭ-ō′pĭ-ă)   Reduced or dim vision

ascites (ă-sī′tēz)   Serous fluid in the peritoneal cavity

asepsis (ā-sĕp′sĭs)   Being free of infection

aspirate (ăs′pĭ-rāte)   To remove by suction

axilla (ăks-ĭl′ă)   Armpit

autopsy (ŏ′tŏp-sē)   Examination of the organs of a dead body to determine the cause of death

biopsy (bī′ŏp-sē)   Section of tissue removed from a living specimen

cataract (căt′ă-răct)   Opacity of the lens of the eye

cerumen (sē-roo′mĕn)   Earwax

cholesterol (kō-lĕs′tĕr-ŏl)   Organic alcohol present in bile, blood, and various tissues

Write each word five times as it is pronounced on the tape.

REVIEW

Fill in the correct term or definition.

1. _afebrile_ without fever
2. **aspirate** _— to remove by suction_
3. _cerumen_ earwax
4. **abscess** _localized coll. of pus in a cavity... tissue_
5. _amblyopia_ reduced or dim vision
6. **biopsy** _section of tissue rem. from a living organism_
7. _cataract_ opacity of lens of the eye
8. **ascites** _serous fluid in the peritoneal c._

Check your answers at the end of the book. If you missed more than one, review Block 1.

Now, proceed with Block 2.

Block 2

These words are pronounced on the tape.

decubitus	epistaxis	insomnia
diaphoresis	exudate	lacrimal
diffuse	flaccid	malaise
diplopia	gangrene	myopia
empyema	hyperpyrexia	

decubitus (dē-kū′bĭ-tŭs)   Bedsore
diaphoresis (dī″ă-fō-rē′sĭs)   Profuse sweating
diffuse (dĭ-fūs′)   Widely scattered
diplopia (dĭp-lō′pĭ-ă)   Double vision
empyema (ĕm″pī-ē′mă)   Pus in a body cavity
epistaxis (ĕp″ĭ-stăk′sĭs)   Nosebleed
exudate (ĕks′ū-dāt)   Accumulation of fluid in a cavity, or the passing out
     of pus or serum
flaccid (flă′sĭd)   Limp, soft
gangrene (găng′grēn)   Death of tissue
hyperpyrexia (hī″pĕr-pī-rĕks′ĭ-ă)   Body temperature greatly above normal
insomnia (ĭn-sŏm′nĭ-ă)   Inability to sleep
lacrimal (lăk′rĭm-ăl)   Pertaining to tears
malaise (mă-lāz′)   Feeling of uneasiness
myopia (mī-ōp′ĭ-ă)   Nearsightedness

REVIEW

Match the following terms with their meanings:

1. diffuse _____   a. soft, limp

2. asepsis _____   b. feeling of uneasiness

3. flaccid _____   c. profuse sweating

4. afebrile _____   d. sharp, sudden

5. hyperpyrexia _____   e. pertaining to tears

6. diaphoresis _____   f. widely scattered

7. malaise _____   g. bedsore

8. acute _____   h. accumulation of fluid in a cavity

9. decubitus _____   i. being free of infection

10. lacrimal _____   j. body temperature greatly above normal

11. exudate _____   k. death of tissue

12. gangrene _____   l. without fever

Check your answers at the end of the book. If you missed more than one, review Blocks 1 and 2.

Block 3

Turn on the tape; the terms are pronounced for you.

palpation	prophylactic	sepsis
palpitation	pruritus	stenosis
petechiae	purulent	tremor
photophobia	pyrexia	ulcer
	sedative	urticaria

palpation (păl-pā′shŭn) Touching with fingers the external surfaces of
   the body to feel the structures beneath
palpitation (păl-pĭ-tā′shŭn) A sensation that one's heart has skipped a
   beat
petechiae (pē-tē′kĭ-ī) Small areas of hemorrhage under the skin
photophobia (fō″tō-fō′bĭ-ă) Hypersensitivity to light
prophylactic (prō-fĭ-lăk′tĭk) Preventive
pruritus (proo-rī′tŭs) Itching
purulent (pūr′ū-lĕnt) Consisting of or containing pus
pyrexia (pī′rĕk′sĭ-ă) Fever
sedative (sĕd′ă-tĭv) Medication producing a quieting effect
sepsis (sĕp′sĭs) An infection or poisoning
stenosis (stĕ-nō′sĭs) Narrowing or constriction of an orifice
tremor (trĕm′ŭr) A trembling
ulcer (ŭl′sĕr) Necrosis, a sore
urticaria (ŭr-tĭ-kā′rĭ-ă) Hives

REVIEW

Fill in the proper term.

palpation	photophobia	palpitation
ulcer	exudate	urticaria
sepsis	diplopia	sedative
epistaxis	pyrexia	myopia
purulent	stenosis	

1. _pyrexia_ fever
2. _photophobia_ hypersensitivity to light
3. _epistaxis_ nosebleed
4. _diplopia_ double vision
5. _urticaria_ hives
6. _ulcer_ necrosis, a sore
7. _stenosis_ narrowing of an orifice
8. _myopia_ nearsightedness
9. _purulent_ containing pus

Check your answers at the end of the book. If you missed more than one, review Blocks 1 through 3.

THESE ARE THE LAST MEDICAL TERMS. GO TO THE INSTRUCTOR FOR TEST NUMBER 8. IT COVERS SECTIONS 12 AND 13. YOU MUST ACHIEVE AT LEAST 80% MASTERY TO PASS.

MEDICAL ABBREVIATIONS

One of the most *confusing* and *useful* parts of medical terminology is the use of abbreviations. Abbreviations are a quick and efficient way of conveying a message. They will be presented to you in a repetitious format, so that you will gradually learn 190 abbreviations.

A set of five abbreviations will be presented at one time. Follow all steps as indicated and review as necessary. After each set of 25 abbreviations are presented and learned, a review is given of those abbreviations.

GOOD LUCK!!

STEP 1. Cover the bottom half of this page.
STEP 2. Study these abbreviations.

āā	Of each, equal parts
abd	Abdomen
ac	Before meals
AD	Right ear
ad lib	As desired

STEP 3. Cover the abbreviations with your hand and try to remember them.
STEP 4. Cover the terms and try to remember them.
STEP 5. Now cover the top of this page and try to write the entire list on scrap paper.
STEP 6. Cover the top half of this page.

STEP 7. Take this check.

1. _____ before meals

2. **āā** _____

3. _____ as desired

4. **AD** _____

5. _____ abdomen

STEP 8. Check your answers on the next page.

ANSWERS

1. **ac**   Before meals
2. **āā**   Of each, equal parts
3. **ad lib**   As desired
4. **AD**   Right ear
5. **abd**   Abdomen

If you did not get all of them correct, go back and practice STEPS 1 through 5. If you did, CONGRATULATIONS! *Now continue.*

STEP 1.   Study these abbreviations.

        adm   Admission
        AK   Above the knee
        AM   Morning
        amb   Ambulate
        amp   Ampule

STEP 2.   Cover the abbreviations with your hand and try to remember them.
STEP 3.   Cover the terms and try to remember them.
STEP 4.   Now cover the whole list and try to write it on scrap paper.

STEP 5. Cover the bottom half of this page.
STEP 6. Take this check.

    1. _____ above the knee

    2. **amp** _____

    3. _____ morning

    4. **adm** _____

    5. _____ ambulate

STEP 7. Uncover the bottom half of this page and check your answers.

ANSWERS

1. **AK** Above the knee
2. **amp** Ampule
3. **AM** Morning
4. **adm** Admission
5. **amb** Ambulate

If you did not get them all correct, go back and practice STEPS 1 through 4. If you did, GREAT! *Now continue.*

STEP 1. Cover the bottom half of this page.
STEP 2. Study these abbreviations.

amt	Amount
AP	Anteroposterior
ARD	Acute respiratory distress
AS	Left ear
ASA	Aspirin

STEP 3. Cover the abbreviations with your hand and try to remember them.
STEP 4. Cover the terms and try to remember them.
STEP 5. Cover the whole list and try to write it on scrap paper.
STEP 6. Cover the top half of this page.

STEP 7. Take this check.

1. _____ anteroposterior

2. **AS** _____

3. _____ aspirin

4. **amt** _____

5. _____ acute respiratory distress

STEP 8. Check your answers on the next page.

ANSWERS

1. **AP** Anteroposterior
2. **AS** Left ear
3. **ASA** Aspirin
4. **amt** Amount
5. **ARD** Acute repiratory distress

If you did not get them all correct, go back and practice STEPS 1 through 5. If you did, GOOD! Now go on.

STEP 1. Study these abbreviations.

as tol	As tolerated
AV	Arteriovenous, atrioventricular
ax	Axillary
BaE	Barium enema
bid	Twice a day

STEP 2. Cover the abbreviations with your hand and try to remember them.

STEP 3. Cover the terms and try to remember them.

STEP 4. Now cover the entire list and try to write it on scrap paper.

STEP 5. Cover the bottom half of this page.
STEP 6. Take this check.

        1. _____ axillary

        2. **AV** _____

        3. _____ as tolerated

        4. **bid** _____

        5. _____ barium enema

STEP 7. Uncover the bottom half of this page and check your answers.

ANSWERS

1. **ax**   axillary
2. **AV**   arteriovenous, atrioventricular
3. **as tol**   As tolerated
4. **bid**   Twice a day
5. **BaE**   Barium enema

If you did not get all of them correct, go back and practice STEPS 1 through 4. If you did, GREAT! *Now continue.*

STEP 1. Cover the bottom half of this page.
STEP 2. Study these abbreviations.

      BMR   Basal metabolic rate
      BP   Blood pressure
      BR   Bed rest
      BRP   Bathroom privileges
      BS   Blood sugar

STEP 3. Cover the abbreviations with your hand and try to remember them.
STEP 4. Cover the terms and try to remember them.
STEP 5. Cover the entire list and try to write it on scrap paper.
STEP 6. Cover the top half of this page.

STEP 7. Take this check.

    1. **BRP** _____

    2. _____ blood pressure

    3. **BMR** _____

    4. _____ bed rest

    5. **BS** _____

STEP 8. Check your answers on the next page.

ANSWERS

1. **BRP** Bathroom privileges
2. **BP** Blood pressure
3. **BMR** Basal metabolic rate
4. **BR** Bed rest
5. **BS** Blood sugar

If you did not get them all correct, go back and practice STEPS 1 through 5. If you did, GOOD! Now go on.

STEP 1. Study the list of 25 abbreviations you have learned.

1. **āā** Of each, equal parts
2. **abd** Abdomen
3. **ac** Before meals
4. **AD** Right ear
5. **ad lib** As desired
6. **adm** Admission
7. **AK** Above the knee
8. **AM** Morning
9. **amb** Ambulate
10. **amp** Ampule
11. **amt** Amount
12. **AP** Anteroposterior
13. **ARD** Acute respiratory distress
14. **AS** Left ear
15. **ASA** Aspirin
16. **as tol** As tolerated
17. **AV** Arteriovenous, atrioventricular
18. **ax** Axillary
19. **BaE** Barium enema
20. **bid** Twice a day
21. **BMR** Basal metabolic rate
22. **BP** Blood pressure
23. **BR** Bed rest
24. **BRP** Bathroom privileges
25. **BS** Blood sugar

STEP 2. Cover up the abbreviations and look at the terms. Try to remember all the abbreviations. Do this until you know all of them.

STEP 3. Next, cover the terms and look at the abbreviations and try to remember all the terms. Do this until you know them all.

STEP 4. Check each term and abbreviation to see if you can spell it properly.

STEP 1. Cover the bottom half of this page.
STEP 2. Study these abbreviations.

BT	Bleeding time
BUN	Blood urea nitrogen
Bx	Biopsy
C	Centigrade
c̄	With

STEP 3. Cover the abbreviations with your hand and try to remember them.
STEP 4. Now cover the terms and try to remember them.
STEP 5. Cover the entire list and try to write it on scrap paper.
STEP 6. Cover the top half of this page.

STEP 7. Take this check.

1. **C** _____

2. _____ bleeding time

3. **Bx** _____

4. _____ with

5. **BUN** _____

STEP 8. Check your answers on the next page.

ANSWERS

1. **C** Centigrade
2. **BT** Bleeding time
3. **Bx** Biopsy
4. **c̄** With
5. **BUN** Blood urea nitrogen

If you did not get all of them correct, go back and practice STEPS 1 through 5. If you did, GOOD! *Go on.*

STEP 1. Study these abbreviations.

CA Carcinoma
Ca⁺⁺ Calcium
cap Capsule
cath Catheter
CBC Complete blood count

STEP 2. Cover the abbreviations with your hand and try to remember them.
STEP 3. Cover the terms and try to remember them.
STEP 4. Cover the whole list and try to write it on scrap paper.

STEP 5. Cover the bottom half of this page.
STEP 6. Take this check.

1. **cath** _____

2. _____ complete blood count

3. **CA** _____

4. _____ calcium

5. **cap** _____

STEP 7. Uncover the bottom half of this page and check your answers.

ANSWERS
1. **cath** Catheter
2. **CBC** Complete blood count
3. **CA** Carcinoma
4. **Ca^{++}** Calcium
5. **cap** Capsule

If you did not get all of them correct, go back and practice STEPS 1 through 4. If you did, TERRIFIC! *Now go on.*

STEP 1. Cover the bottom half of this page.
STEP 2. Study these abbreviations.

CC   Chief complaint
CHD   Congenital heart disease
chr   Chronic
Cl   Chloride
CNS   Central nervous system

STEP 3. Cover the abbreviations with your hand and try to remember them.
STEP 4. Cover the terms and try to remember them.
STEP 5. Now cover the whole list and try to write it on scrap paper.
STEP 6. Cover the top half of this page.

STEP 7. Take this check.

1. **chr** _____

2. _____ central nervous system

3. **CHD** _____

4. _____ chief complaint

5. **Cl** _____

STEP 8. Check your answers on the next page.

ANSWERS

1. **chr**   Chronic
2. **CNS**   Central nervous system
3. **CHD**   Congenital heart disease
4. **CC**   Chief complaint
5. **Cl**   Chloride

If you did not get all of them correct, go back and practice STEPS 1 through 5. If you did, GOOD! *Now continue.*

STEP 1. Study these abbreviations.

CO_2	Carbon dioxide
COPD	Chronic obstructive pulmonary disease
C-section	Cesarean section
CSF	Cerebrospinal fluid
cu mm	Cubic millimeter

STEP 2. Cover the abbreviations with your hand and try to remember them.

STEP 3. Cover the terms and try to remember them.

STEP 4. Cover the entire list and try to write it on scrap paper.

STEP 5. Cover the bottom half of this page.
STEP 6. Take this check.

       1. _____ cubic millimeter

       2. **CSF** _____

       3. _____ carbon dioxide

       4. **COPD** _____

       5. _____ cesarean section

STEP 7. Uncover the bottom half of this page and check your answers.

ANSWERS
1. **cu mm** Cubic millimeter
2. **CSF** Cerebrospinal fluid
3. **CO_2** Carbon dioxide
4. **COPD** Chronic obstructive pulmonary disease
5. **C-section** Cesarean section

*If you did not get all of them correct, go back and review STEPS 1
through 4. If you did,* GOOD! *Now continue.*

STEP 1. Cover the bottom half of this page.
STEP 2. Study these abbreviations.

CVA   Cerebrovascular accident
CXR   Chest x-ray
cysto Cystoscopy
DAT   Diet as tolerated
DC   Discontinue

STEP 3. Cover the abbreviations with your hand and try to remember them.
STEP 4. Cover the terms and try to remember them.
STEP 5. Cover the whole list and try to write it on scrap paper.
STEP 6. Cover the top half of this page.

STEP 7. Take this check.

1. **DC** _____

2. _____ chest x-ray

3. **CVA** _____

4. _____ cystoscopy

5. **DAT** _____

STEP 8. Check your answers on the next page.

ANSWERS
1. **DC**   Discontinue
2. **CXR**   Chest x-ray
3. **CVA**   Cerebrovascular accident
4. **cysto**   Cystoscopy
5. **DAT**   Diet as tolerated

If you did not get all of them correct, go back and practice STEPS 1 through 5. If you did, GREAT! *Now continue.*

STEP 1. Study the 50 abbreviations you have learned so far.

1.	**āā**	Of each, equal parts
2.	**abd**	Abdomen
3.	**ac**	Before meals
4.	**AD**	Right ear
5.	**ad lib**	As desired
6.	**adm**	Admission
7.	**AK**	Above the knee
8.	**AM**	Morning
9.	**amb**	Ambulate
10.	**amp**	Ampule
11.	**amt**	Amount
12.	**AP**	Anteroposterior
13.	**ARD**	Acute respiratory distress
14.	**AS**	Left ear
15.	**ASA**	Aspirin
16.	**as tol**	As tolerated
17.	**AV**	Arteriovenous, atrioventricular
18.	**ax**	Axillary
19.	**BaE**	Barium enema
20.	**bid**	Twice a day
21.	**BMR**	Basal metabolic rate
22.	**BP**	Blood pressure
23.	**BR**	Bed rest
24.	**BRP**	Bathroom privileges
25.	**BS**	Blood sugar
26.	**BT**	Bleeding time
27.	**BUN**	Blood urea nitrogen
28.	**Bx**	Biopsy
29.	**C**	Centigrade
30.	**c̄**	With

31.	**CA**	Carcinoma
32.	**CA^{++}**	Calcium
33.	**cap**	Capsule
34.	**cath**	Catheter
35.	**CBC**	Complete blood count
36.	**CC**	Chief complaint
37.	**CHD**	Congenital heart disease
38.	**chr**	Chronic
39.	**Cl**	Chloride
40.	**CNS**	Central nervous system
41.	**CO$_2$**	Carbon dioxide
42.	**COPD**	Chronic obstructive pulmonary disease
43.	**C-section**	Cesarean section
44.	**CSF**	Cerebrospinal fluid
45.	**cu mm**	Cubic millimeter
46.	**CVA**	Cerebrovascular accident
47.	**CXR**	Chest x-ray
48.	**cysto**	Cystoscopy
49.	**DAT**	Diet as tolerated
50.	**DC**	Discontinue

STEP 2. Cover the abbreviations and look at the terms. Try to remember all of the abbreviations. Do the same with the terms, and do this until you know them all. Be careful of the spelling.

STEP 3. Take this check.

     1. **AS** _____

     2. _____ centigrade

     3. **chr** _____

     4. **BMR** _____

     5. _____ diet as tolerated

     6. _____ carbon dioxide

     7. **BUN** _____

     8. _____ chloride

     9. **AV** _____

   10. **ad lib** _____

   11. **AD** _____

   12. **CVA** _____

   13. _____ cerebrospinal fluid

   14. _____ biopsy

   15. **ARD** _____

   16. _____ catheter

   17. **bid** _____

   18. **ASA** _____

   19. _____ barium enema

   20. _____ discontinue

STEP 4. Check your answers on the next page.

ANSWERS

1. **AS** Left ear
2. **C** Centigrade
3. **chr** Chronic
4. **BMR** Basal metabolic rate
5. **DAT** Diet as tolerated
6. **CO_2** Carbon dioxide
7. **BUN** Blood urea nitrogen
8. **Cl** Chloride
9. **AV** Arteriovenous, atrioventricular
10. **ad lib** As desired
11. **AD** Right ear
12. **CVA** Cerebrovascular accident
13. **CSF** Cerebrospinal fluid
14. **Bx** Biopsy
15. **ARD** Acute respiratory distress
16. **cath** Catheter
17. **bid** Twice a day
18. **ASA** Aspirin
19. **BaE** Barium enema
20. **DC** Discontinue

If you missed more than two, repeat STEP 1. It is important for you to know the first 50 abbreviations before continuing. If you got them all correct, GREAT! *Continue.*

STEP 1. Cover the bottom half of this page.
STEP 2. Study these abbreviations.

D & C	Dilation and curettage
diag, Dx	Diagnosis
diff	Differential white blood count
DM	Diabetes mellitus
DOB	Date of birth

STEP 3. Cover the abbreviations with your hand and try to remember them.
STEP 4. Cover the terms and try to remember them.
STEP 5. Cover the whole list and try to write it on scrap paper.
STEP 6. Cover the top half of this page.

STEP 7. Take this check.

1. **DM** _____

2. **Dx** _____

3. _____ date of birth

4. _____ differential white blood count

5. **D & C** _____

STEP 8. Check your answers on the next page.

ANSWERS
1. **DM**   Diabetes mellitus
2. **Dx**   Diagnosis
3. **DOB**   Date of birth
4. **diff**   Differential white blood count
5. **D & C**   Dilation and curettage

If you did not get all of them correct, go back and practice STEPS 1 through 5. If you did, TERRIFIC! Go on.

STEP 1. Study these abbreviations.

dr, ʒ	Dram
DT	Delirium tremens
DUB	Dysfunctional uterine bleeding
EEG	Electroencephalogram
EENT	Eyes, ears, nose, throat

STEP 2. Cover the abbreviations with your hand and try to remember them.

STEP 3. Now cover the terms and try to remember them.

STEP 4. Cover the whole list and try to write it on scrap paper.

STEP 5. Cover the bottom half of this page.
STEP 6. Take this check.

      1. **EEG** _____

      2. **DUB** _____

      3. _____ dram

      4. _____ delirium tremens

      5. **EENT** _____

STEP 7. Uncover the bottom half of this page and check your answers.

ANSWERS
1. **EEG** Electroencephalogram
2. **DUB** Dysfunctional uterine bleeding
3. **Dr, 3** Dram
4. **DT** Delirium tremens
5. **EENT** Eye, ear, nose, throat

If you did not get all of them correct, go back and practice STEPS 1 through 4. If not, VERY GOOD! _Now go on._

STEP 1. Cover the bottom half of this page.
STEP 2. Study these abbreviations.

EKG	Electrocardiogram
elix	Elixir
EMG	Electromyogram
ER	Emergency room
exc	Excision

STEP 3. Cover the abbreviations with your hand and try to remember them.
STEP 4. Cover the terms and try to remember them.
STEP 5. Cover the entire list and try to write it on scrap paper.
STEP 6. Cover the top half of this page.

STEP 7. Take this check.

1. **exc** _____

2. _____ emergency room

3. _____ electrocardiogram

4. **EMG** _____

5. **elix** _____

Step 8. Check your answers on the next page.

ANSWERS

1. **exc**   Excision
2. **ER**   Emergency room
3. **EKG**   Electrocardiogram
4. **EMG**   Electromyogram
5. **elix**   Elixir

If you did not get all of them correct, go back and practice STEPS 1 through 5. If you did, YOU'RE DOING FINE! *Now go on.*

STEP 1. Study these abbreviations.

F	Fahrenheit
FBS	Fasting blood sugar
FDA	Food and Drug Administration
Fe	Iron
FH	Family history

STEP 2. Cover the abbreviations with your hand and try to remember them.

STEP 3. Cover the terms and try to remember them.

STEP 4. Cover the entire list and try to write it on scrap paper.

STEP 5. Cover the bottom half of this page.
STEP 6. Take this check.

      1. **FDA** _____

      2. _____ iron

      3. **FH** _____

      4. **FBS** _____

      5. _____ Fahrenheit

STEP 7. Uncover the bottom half of this page and check your answers.

ANSWERS

1. **FDA** Food and Drug Administration
2. **Fe** Iron
3. **FH** Family history
4. **FBS** Fasting blood sugar
5. **F** Fahrenheit

If you did not get all of them correct, go back and practice STEPS 1 through 4. If you did, GOOD! Continue.

STEP 1. Cover the bottom half of this page.
STEP 2. Study these abbreviations.

FHT	Fetal heart tone
FSH	Follicle-stimulating hormone
FUO	Fever of undetermined origin
GB	Gallbladder
GBS	Gallbladder series

STEP 3. Cover the abbreviations with your hand and try to remember them.
STEP 4. Cover the terms and try to remember them.
STEP 5. Cover the entire list and try to write it on scrap paper.
STEP 6. Cover the top half of this page.

STEP 7. Take this check.

1. **FHT** _____

2. **GBS** _____

3. _____ gallbladder

4. **FSH** _____

5. **FUO** _____

STEP 8. Check your answers on the next page.

ANSWERS

1. **FHT**   Fetal heart tone
2. **GBS**   Gallbladder series
3. **GB**   Gallbladder
4. **FSH**   Follicle-stimulating hormone
5. **FUO**   Fever of undetermined origin

If you missed any, go back and practice STEPS 1 through 5. If not, TERRIFIC! *Now continue.*

STEP 1. Study the 75 abbreviations you should know.

1. **āā**   Of each, equal parts
2. **abd**   Abdomen
3. **ac**   Before meals
4. **AD**   Right ear
5. **ad lib**   As desired
6. **adm**   Admission
7. **AK**   Above the knee
8. **AM**   Morning
9. **amb**   Ambulate
10. **amp**   Ampule
11. **amt**   Amount
12. **AP**   Anteroposterior
13. **ARD**   Acute respiratory distress
14. **AS**   Left ear
15. **ASA**   Aspirin
16. **as tol**   As tolerated
17. **AV**   Arteriovenous, atrioventricular
18. **ax**   Axillary
19. **BaE**   Barium enema
20. **bid**   Twice a day
21. **BMR**   Basal metabolic rate
22. **BP**   Blood pressure
23. **BR**   Bed rest
24. **BRP**   Bathroom privileges
25. **BS**   Blood sugar
26. **BT**   Bleeding time
27. **BUN**   Blood urea nitrogen
28. **Bx**   Biopsy
29. **C**   Centigrade
30. **c̄**   With
31. **CA**   Carcinoma
32. **Ca^{++}** Calcium
33. **cap**   Capsule

34.	**cath**	Catheter
35.	**CBC**	Complete blood count
36.	**CC**	Chief complaint
37.	**CHD**	Congenital heart disease
38.	**chr**	Chronic
39.	**Cl**	Chloride
40.	**CNS**	Central nervous system
41.	**CO$_2$**	Carbon dioxide
42.	**COPD**	Chronic obstructive pulmonary disease
43.	**C-section**	Cesarean section
44.	**CSF**	Cerebrospinal fluid
45.	**cu mm**	Cubic millimeter
46.	**CVA**	Cerebrovascular accident
47.	**CXR**	Chest x-ray
48.	**cysto**	Cystoscopy
49.	**DAT**	Diet as tolerated
50.	**DC**	Discontinue
51.	**D & C**	Dilation and curettage
52.	**diag, DX**	Diagnosis
53.	**diff**	Differential white blood count
54.	**DM**	Diabetes mellitus
55.	**DOB**	Date of birth
56.	**dr, $_3$**	Dram
57.	**DT**	Delirium tremens
58.	**DUB**	Dysfunctional uterine bleeding
59.	**EEG**	Electroencephalogram
60.	**EENT**	Eye, ear, nose, throat
61.	**EKG**	Electrocardiogram
62.	**elix**	Elixir
63.	**EMG**	Electromyogram
64.	**ER**	Emergency room
65.	**exc**	Excision
66.	**F**	Fahrenheit
67.	**FBS**	Fasting blood sugar
68.	**FDA**	Food and Drug Administration
69.	**Fe**	Iron
70.	**FH**	Family history
71.	**FHT**	Fetal heart tone
72.	**FSH**	Follicle-stimulating hormone
73.	**FUO**	Fever of undetermined origin
74.	**GB**	Gallbladder
75.	**GBS**	Gallbladder series

STEP 2. Cover the abbreviations and look at the terms. Try to remember them. Do the same with the terms. Do this until you know them all. Check carefully for correct spelling.

STEP 3. Take this check.

    1. _____ with

    2. _____ iron

    3. _____ calcium

    4. _____ dram

    5. **ASA** _____

    6. **FBS** _____

    7. _____ excision

    8. **DT** _____

    9. _____ ampule

   10. **CBC** _____

   11. _____ diagnosis

   12. **FHT** _____

   13. **elix** _____

   14. **DOB** _____

   15. _____ blood sugar

   16. **BT** _____

   17. _____ above the knee

   18. **COPD** _____

   19. _____ electrocardiogram

   20. **FH** _____

STEP 4. Check your answers on the next page.

ANSWERS

1. **c̄** with
2. **Fe** iron
3. **Ca^{++}** Calcium
4. **dr, ʒ** dram
5. **ASA** Aspirin
6. **FBS** Fasting blood sugar
7. **exc** excision
8. **DT** Delirium tremens
9. **amp** ampule
10. **CBC** Complete blood count
11. **diag, Dx** diagnosis
12. **FHT** Fetal heart tone
13. **elix** Elixir
14. **DOB** Date of birth
15. **BS** Blood sugar
16. **BT** Bleeding time
17. **AK** Above the knee
18. **COPD** Chronic obstructive pulmonary disease
19. **EKG** Electrocardiogram
20. **FH** Family history

If you missed more than two, review STEP 1. If not, SUPER! *Continue.*

STEP 1. Cover the bottom half of this page.
STEP 2. Study these abbreviations.

Gc	Gonorrhea
GI	Gastrointestinal
gm	Gram
gr	Grain
GTT	Glucose tolerance test

STEP 3. Cover the abbreviations with your hand and try to remember them.
STEP 4. Cover the terms and try to remember them.
STEP 5. Cover the entire list and try to write it on scrap paper.
STEP 6. Cover the top half of this page.

STEP 7. Take this check.

1. **gr** _____

2. _____ glucose tolerance test

3. **GI** _____

4. **Gc** _____

5. _____ gram

STEP 7. Check your answers on the next page.

ANSWERS
1. **gr** Grain
2. **GTT** Glucose tolerance test
3. **GI** Gastrointestinal
4. **Gc** Gonorrhea
5. **gm** Gram

If you missed any, review STEPS 1 through 5. If not, VERY GOOD! *Now continue.*

STEP 1. Study these abbreviations.

gtt	Drop
Gyn	Gynecology
HCl	Hydrochloric acid
Hct	Hematocrit
Hgb	Hemoglobin

STEP 2. Cover the abbreviations with your hand and try to remember them.

STEP 3. Cover the terms and try to remember them.

STEP 4. Cover the entire list and try to write it on scrap paper.

STEP 5. Cover the bottom half of this page.
STEP 6. Take this check.

1. _____ hematocrit

2. **HCl** _____

3. **Gyn** _____

4. _____ hemoglobin

5. **gtt** _____

STEP 7. Uncover the bottom half of this page and check your answers.

ANSWERS
1. **Hct** Hematocrit
2. **HCl** Hydrochloric acid
3. **Gyn** Gynecology
4. **Hgb** Hemoglobin
5. **gtt** Drop

If you missed any abbreviations, go back and review STEPS 1 through 4.
If you did not, KEEP UP THE GOOD WORK! *Continue.*

STEP 1. Cover the bottom half of this page.
STEP 2. Study these abbreviations.

> H_2O Water
> H_2O_2 Hydrogen peroxide
> H & P   History and physical
> hs   Hour of sleep
> HVD   Hypertensive vascular disease

STEP 3. Cover the abbreviations with your hand and try to remember them.
STEP 4. Cover the terms and try to remember them.
STEP 5. Cover the whole list and try to write it on scrap paper.
STEP 6. Cover the top half of this page.

STEP 7. Take this check.

1. _____ hour of sleep

2. H_2O_2 _____

3. _____ history and physical

4. H_2O _____

5. HVD _____

STEP 8. Check your answers on the next page.

ANSWERS

1. **hs**   Hour of sleep
2. **H₂O₂**   Hydrogen peroxide
3. **H & P**   History and physical
4. **H₂O**   Water
5. **HVD**   Hypertensive vascular disease

If you missed any, go back and practice STEPS 1 through 5. If all were correct, GREAT! *Now go on.*

STEP 1. Study these abbreviations.

Hx	History
hypo	Hypodermic injection
I^{131}	Radioactive iodine
IM	Intramuscular
inf	Infusion

STEP 2. Cover the abbreviations with your hand and try to remember them.

STEP 3. Cover the terms and try to remember them.

STEP 4. Cover the entire list and try to write it on scrap paper.

STEP 5. Cover the bottom half of this page.
STEP 6. Take this check.

1. **inf** _____

2. _____ radioactive iodine

3. _____ hypodermic injection

4. _____ history

5. **IM** _____

STEP 7. Uncover the bottom half of this page and check your answers.

ANSWERS
1. **inf**   Infusion
2. I^{131} Radioactive iodine
3. **hypo**   Hypodermic injection
4. **Hx**   History
5. **IM**   Intramuscular

If you missed any, go back and practice STEPS 1 through 4. If all were correct, go on.

STEP 1. Cover the bottom half of this page.
STEP 2. Study these abbreviations.

inj   Injection
IPPB Intermittent positive pressure breathing
IQ   Intelligence quotient
IUD   Intrauterine device
IV   Intravenous

STEP 3. Cover the abbreviations with your hand and try to remember them.
STEP 4. Cover the terms and try to remember them.
STEP 5. Cover the entire list and try to write it on scrap paper.
STEP 6. Cover the top half of this page.

STEP 7. Take this check.

1. **IUD** _____

2. _____ injection

3. **IPPB** _____

4. _____ intravenous

5. **IQ** _____

STEP 8. Check your answers on the next page.

ANSWERS

1. **IUD**   Intrauterine device
2. **inj**   Injection
3. **IPPB**   Intermittent positive pressure breathing
4. **IV**   Intravenous
5. **IQ**   Intelligence quotient

*If you did not get all of them correct, go back and review STEPS 1
through 5. If all were correct,* FANTASTIC! *Go on.*

STEP 1. Study the 100 abbreviations you should know.

1.	āā	Of each, equal parts
2.	abd	Abdomen
3.	ac	Before meals
4.	AD	Right ear
5.	ad lib	As desired
6.	adm	Admission
7.	AK	Above the knee
8.	AM	Morning
9.	amb	Ambulate
10.	amp	Ampule
11.	amt	Amount
12.	AP	Anteroposterior
13.	ARD	Acute respiratory distress
14.	AS	Left ear
15.	ASA	Aspirin
16.	as tol	As tolerated
17.	AV	Arteriovenous, atrioventricular
18.	ax	Axillary
19.	BaE	Barium enema
20.	bid	Twice a day
21.	BMR	Basal metabolic rate
22.	BP	Blood pressure
23.	BR	Bed rest
24.	BRP	Bathroom privileges
25.	BS	Blood sugar
26.	BT	Bleeding time
27.	BUN	Blood urea nitrogen
28.	Bx	Biopsy
29.	C	Centigrade
30.	c̄	With
31.	CA	Carcinoma
32.	Ca^{++}	Calcium

33.	**cap**	Capsule
34.	**cath**	Catheter
35.	**CBC**	Complete blood count
36.	**CC**	Chief complaint
37.	**CHD**	Congenital heart disease
38.	**chr**	Chronic
39.	**Cl**	Chloride
40.	**CNS**	Central nervous system
41.	**CO$_2$**	Carbon dioxide
42.	**COPD**	Chronic obstructive pulmonary disease
43.	**C-section**	Cesarean section
44.	**CSF**	Cerebrospinal fluid
45.	**cu mm**	Cubic millimeter
46.	**CVA**	Cerebrovascular accident
47.	**CXR**	Chest x-ray
48.	**cysto**	Cystoscopy
49.	**DAT**	Diet as tolerated
50.	**DC**	Discontinue
51.	**D & C**	Dilation and curettage
52.	**diag, Dx**	Diagnosis
53.	**diff**	Differential white blood count
54.	**DM**	Diabetes mellitus
55.	**DOB**	Date of birth
56.	**dr, ʒ**	Dram
57.	**DT**	Delirium tremens
58.	**DUB**	Dysfunctional uterine bleeding
59.	**EEG**	Electroencephalogram
60.	**EENT**	Eye, ear, nose, throat
61.	**EKG**	Electrocardiogram
62.	**elix**	Elixir
63.	**EMG**	Electromyogram
64.	**ER**	Emergency room
65.	**exc**	Excision
66.	**F**	Fahrenheit
67.	**FBS**	Fasting blood sugar
68.	**FDA**	Food and Drug Administration
69.	**Fe**	Iron
70.	**FH**	Family history
71.	**FHT**	Fetal heart tone
72.	**FSH**	Follicle-stimulating hormone
73.	**FUO**	Fever of undetermined origin
74.	**GB**	Gallbladder
75.	**GBS**	Gallbladder series
76.	**Gc**	Gonorrhea
77.	**GI**	Gastrointestinal

78. **gm**   Gram
79. **gr**   Grain
80. **GTT**   Glucose tolerance test
81. **gtt**   Drop
82. **Gyn**   Gynecology
83. **HCl**   Hydrochloric acid
84. **Hct**   Hematocrit
85. **Hgb**   Hemoglobin
86. **H_2O**   Water
87. **H_2O_2**   Hydrogen peroxide
88. **H & P**   History and physical
89. **hs**   Hour of sleep
90. **HVD**   Hypertensive vascular disease
91. **Hx**   History
92. **hypo**   Hypodermic injection
93. **I^{131}**   Radioactive iodine
94. **IM**   Intramuscular
95. **inf**   Infusion
96. **inj**   Injection
97. **IPPB**   Intermittent positive pressure breathing
98. **IQ**   Intelligence quotient
99. **IUD**   Intrauterine device
100. **IV**   Intravenous

STEP 2. Take this check.

1. _____ radioactive iodine

2. _____ hour of sleep

3. **cu mm** _____

4. _____ grain

5. _____ fever of undetermined origin

6. _____ hemoglobin

7. **CHD** _____

8. _____ drop

9. _____ ambulate

10. **āā** _____

11. _____ history

12. _____ gonorrhea

13. **DM** _____

14. **CXR** _____

15. _____ hydrogen peroxide

16. **IQ** _____

17. _____ gram

18. **EEG** _____

19. **CC** _____

20. _____ glucose tolerance test

21. **HVD** _____

22. **ac** _____

23. _____ hematocrit

24. _____ carcinoma

25. **EMG** _____

STEP 3. Check your answers on the next page.

ANSWERS

1. I^{131} Radioactive iodine
2. **hs**   Hour of sleep
3. **cu mm**   Cubic millimeter
4. **gr**   Grain
5. **FUO**   Fever of undetermined origin
6. **Hgb**   Hemoglobin
7. **CHD**   Congenital heart disease
8. **gtt**   Drop
9. **amb**   Ambulate
10. **āā**   Of each, equal parts
11. **Hx**   History
12. **Gc**   Gonorrhea
13. **DM**   Diabetes mellitus
14. **CXR**   Chest x-ray
15. **H_2O_2**   Hydrogen peroxide
16. **IQ**   Intelligence quotient
17. **gm**   Gram
18. **EEG**   Electroencephalogram
19. **CC**   Chief complaint
20. **GTT**   Glucose tolerance test
21. **HVD**   Hypertensive vascular disease
22. **ac**   Before meals
23. **Hct**   Hematocrit
24. **CA**   Carcinoma
25. **EMG**   Electromyogram

If you missed more than two, thoroughly review STEP 1. If not, so far so good. Continue.

STEP 1. Cover the bottom half of this page.
STEP 2. Study these abbreviations.

IVP	Intravenous pyelogram
K$^+$	Potassium
kg	Kilogram
KUB	Kidney, ureter, bladder
KVO	Keep vein open

STEP 3. Cover the abbreviations with your hand and try to remember them.
STEP 4. Cover the terms and try to remember them.
STEP 5. Cover the entire list and try to write it on scrap paper.
STEP 6. Cover the top half of this page.

STEP 7. Take this check.

1. **KUB** _____

2. _____ potassium

3. **KVO** _____

4. **IVP** _____

5. _____ kilogram

STEP 8. Check your answers on the next page.

ANSWERS

1. **KUB** Kidney, ureter, bladder
2. **K⁺** Potassium
3. **KVO** Keep vein open
4. **IVP** Intravenous pyelogram
5. **kg** Kilogram

If you did not get them all correct, go back and review STEPS 1 through 5. If all were correct, YOU'RE DOING FINE! *Continue.*

STEP 1. Study these abbreviations.

L	Liter, left, lumbar spine
lab	Laboratory
lb	Pound
liq	Liquid
LKS	Liver, kidney, spleen

STEP 2. Cover the abbreviations with your hand and try to remember them.

STEP 3. Cover the terms and try to remember them.

STEP 4. Cover the entire list and try to write it on scrap paper.

STEP 5. Cover the bottom half of this page.
STEP 6. Take this check.

1. **LKS** _____

2. _____ liquid

3. **L** _____

4. **lab** _____

5. _____ pound

STEP 7. Uncover the bottom half of this page and check your answers.

ANSWERS
1. **LKS**   Liver, kidney, spleen
2. **liq**   Liquid
3. **L**   Liter, left, lumbar spine
4. **lab**   Laboratory
5. **lb**   Pound

If you did not get them all correct, review STEPS 1 through 4. If you did,
VERY GOOD! *Continue.*

STEP 1. Cover the bottom half of this page.
STEP 2. Study these abbreviations.

      LLL   Left lower lobe (lung)
      LLQ Left lower quadrant (abd)
      LMP Last menstrual period
      LOC Level of consciousness
      LUL Left upper lobe (lung)

STEP 3. Cover the abbreviations with your hand and try to remember them.
STEP 4. Cover the terms and try to remember them.
STEP 5. Cover the entire list and try to write it on scrap paper.
STEP 6. Cover the top half of this page.

STEP 7. Take this check.

    1. _____ left lower lobe (lung)

    2. **LLQ** _____

    3. **LMP** _____

    4. _____ left upper lobe (lung)

    5. **LOC** _____

STEP 8. Check your answers on the next page.

ANSWERS
1. **LLL**   Left lower lobe (lung)
2. **LLQ**   Left lower quadrant (abd)
3. **LMP**   Last menstrual period
4. **LUL**   Left upper lobe (lung)
5. **LOC**   Level of consciousness

If you did not get all of them correct, review STEPS 1 through 5. If all were correct, KEEP UP THE GOOD WORK! *Now go on.*

STEP 1. Study these abbreviations.

LUQ	Left upper quadrant (abd)
L & W	Living and well
mEq	Milliequivalent
Mg^{++}	Magnesium
mg	Milligram

STEP 2. Cover the abbreviations with your hand and try to remember them.
STEP 3. Cover the terms and try to remember them.
STEP 4. Cover the entire list and try to write it on scrap paper.

STEP 5. Cover the bottom half of this page.
STEP 6. Take this check.

1. _____ milliequivalent

2. **LUQ** _____

3. _____ magnesium

4. **L & W** _____

5. _____ milligram

STEP 7. Uncover the bottom half of this page and check your answers.

ANSWERS

1. **mEq** Milliequivalent
2. **LUQ** Left upper quadrant (abd)
3. **Mg^{++}** Magnesium
4. **L & W** Living and well
5. **mg** Milligram

If you did not get all of them correct, go back and practice STEPS 1 through 4. If you did get them all correct, continue.

STEP 1. Cover the bottom half of this page.
STEP 2. Study these abbreviations.

MI	Myocardial infarction
mm	millimeter
Mn^{--}	Manganese
Na^{+}	Sodium
NaCl	Sodium chloride

STEP 3. Cover the abbreviations and try to remember them.
STEP 4. Cover the terms and try to remember them.
STEP 5. Cover the entire list and try to write it on scrap paper.
STEP 6. Cover the top half of this page.

STEP 7. Take this check.

1. _____ manganese

2. **Na**$^{+}$ _____

3. **MI** _____

4. _____ millimeter

5. **NaCl** _____

STEP 8. Check your answers on the next page.

ANSWERS

1. **Mn^{--}** Manganese
2. **Na$^+$** Sodium
3. **MI** Myocardial infarction
4. **mm** Millimeter
5. **NaCl** Sodium chloride

If you did not get all of them correct, review STEPS 1 through 5. If you did, GOOD! *Now, continue.*

STEP 1. Study the 125 abbreviations you should know.

1.	**āā**	Of each, equal parts
2.	**abd**	Abdomen
3.	**ac**	Before meals
4.	**AD**	Right ear
5.	**ad lib**	As desired
6.	**adm**	Admission
7.	**AK**	Above the knee
8.	**AM**	Morning
9.	**amb**	Ambulate
10.	**amp**	Ampule
11.	**amt**	Amount
12.	**AP**	Anteroposterior
13.	**ARD**	Acute respiratory distress
14.	**AS**	Left ear
15.	**ASA**	Aspirin
16.	**as tol**	As tolerated
17.	**AV**	Arteriovenous, atrioventricular
18.	**ax**	Axillary
19.	**BaE**	Barium enema
20.	**bid**	Twice a day
21.	**BMR**	Basal metabolic rate
22.	**BP**	Blood pressure
23.	**BR**	Bed rest
24.	**BRP**	Bathroom privileges
25.	**BS**	Blood sugar
26.	**BT**	Bleeding time
27.	**BUN**	Blood urea nitrogen
28.	**Bx**	Biopsy
29.	**C**	Centigrade
30.	**c̄**	With
31.	**CA**	Carcinoma
32.	**Ca^{++}**	Calcium
33.	**cap**	Capsule

34. **cath**   Catheter
35. **CBC**   Complete blood count
36. **CC**   Chief complaint
37. **CHD**   Congenital heart disease
38. **chr**   Chronic
39. **Cl**   Chloride
40. **CNS**   Central nervous system
41. **CO$_2$**   Carbon dioxide
42. **COPD**   Chronic obstructive pulmonary disease
43. **C-section** Cesarean section
44. **CSF**   Cerebrospinal fluid
45. **cu mm**   Cubic millimeter
46. **CVA**   Cerebrovascular accident
47. **CXR**   Chest x-ray
48. **cysto**   Cystoscopy
49. **DAT**   Diet as tolerated
50. **DC**   Discontinue
51. **D & C**   Dilation and curettage
52. **diag, Dx**   Diagnosis
53. **diff**   Differential white blood count
54. **DM**   Diabetes mellitus
55. **DOB**   Date of birth
56. **dr, 3**   Dram
57. **DT**   Delirium tremens
58. **DUB**   Dysfunctional uterine bleeding
59. **EEG**   Electroencephalogram
60. **EENT**   Eye, ear, nose, throat
61. **EKG**   Electrocardiogram
62. **elix**   Elixir
63. **EMG**   Electromyogram
64. **ER**   Emergency room
65. **exc**   Excision
66. **F**   Fahrenheit
67. **FBS**   Fasting blood sugar
68. **FDA**   Food and Drug Administration
69. **Fe**   Iron
70. **FH**   Family history
71. **FHT**   Fetal heart tone
72. **FSH**   Follicle-stimulating hormone
73. **FUO**   Fever of undetermined origin
74. **GB**   Gallbladder
75. **GBS**   Gallbladder series
76. **Gc**   Gonorrhea
77. **GI**   Gastrointestinal
78. **gm**   Gram
79. **gr**   Grain

80.	**GTT**	Glucose tolerance test
81.	**gtt**	Drop
82.	**Gyn**	Gynecology
83.	**HCl**	Hydrochloric acid
84.	**Hct**	Hematocrit
85.	**Hgb**	Hemoglobin
86.	**H_2O**	Water
87.	**H_2O_2**	Hydrogen peroxide
88.	**H & P**	History and physical
89.	**hs**	Hour of sleep
90.	**HVD**	Hypertensive vascular disease
91.	**Hx**	History
92.	**hypo**	Hypodermic injection
93.	**I^{131}**	Radioactive iodine
94.	**IM**	Intramuscular
95.	**inf**	Infusion
96.	**inj**	Injection
97.	**IPPB**	Intermittent positive pressure breathing
98.	**IQ**	Intelligence quotient
99.	**IUD**	Intrauterine device
100.	**IV**	Intravenous
101.	**IVP**	Intravenous pyelogram
102.	**K^+**	Potassium
103.	**kg**	Kilogram
104.	**KUB**	Kidney, ureter, bladder
105.	**KVO**	Keep vein open
106.	**L**	Liter, left, lumbar spine
107.	**lab**	Laboratory
108.	**lb**	Pound
109.	**liq**	Liquid
110.	**LKS**	Liver, kidney, spleen
111.	**LLL**	Left lower lobe (lung)
112.	**LLQ**	Left lower quadrant (abd)
113.	**LMP**	Last menstrual period
114.	**LOC**	Level of consciousness
115.	**LUL**	Left upper lobe (lung)
116.	**LUQ**	Left upper quadrant (abd)
117.	**L & W**	Living and well
118.	**mEq**	Milliequivalent
119.	**Mg^{++}**	Magnesium
120.	**mg**	Milligram
121.	**MI**	Myocardial infarction
122.	**mm**	Millimeter
123.	**Mn^{--}**	Manganese
124.	**Na^+**	Sodium
125.	**NaCl**	Sodium chloride

STEP 2. Take this check.

1. **L & W** _____

2. _____ milliequivalent

3. **LKS** _____

4. _____ intelligence quotient

5. **Na$^+$** _____

6. _____ gonorrhea

7. **Hgb** _____

8. _____ dram

9. **ac** _____

10. _____ anteroposterior

11. **H$_2$O$_2$** _____

12. **I^{131}** _____

13. _____ manganese

14. **CXR** _____

15. _____ centigrade

16. **LKS** _____

17. _____ hour of sleep

18. **K$^+$** _____

19. _____ kilogram

20. _____ water

21. **mm** _____

22. **LLL** _____

23. _____ keep vein open

24. **COPD** _____

25. _____ left ear

STEP 3. Check your answers on the next page.

ANSWERS

1. **L & W**   Living and well
2. **mEq**   milliequivalent
3. **LKS**   Liver, kidney, spleen
4. **IQ**   Intelligence quotient
5. **Na^{++}**   Sodium
6. **Gc**   Gonorrhea
7. **Hgb**   Hemoglobin
8. **dr, $\mathfrak{z}$**   Dram
9. **ac**   Before meals
10. **AP**   Anteroposterior
11. **H_2O_2**   Hydrogen peroxide
12. **I^{131}**   Radioactive iodine
13. **Mn^{--}**   Manganese
14. **CXR**   Chest x-ray
15. **C**   Centigrade
16. **LKS**   Liver, kidney, spleen
17. **hs**   Hour of sleep
18. **K$^+$**   Potassium
19. **kg**   Kilogram
20. **H_2O**   Water
21. **mm**   Millimeter
22. **LLL**   Left lower lobe (lung)
23. **KVO**   Keep vein open
24. **COPD**   Chronic obstructive pulmonary disease
25. **AS**   Left ear

If you missed more than two, review STEP 1. It is essential that you learn these abbreviations before continuing in the text. If you did not miss any, GREAT, go on.

STEP 1. Cover the bottom half of this page.
STEP 2. Study these abbreviations.

NB	Newborn
neg	Negative
NG	Nasogastric
NPO	Nothing by mouth
N/S	Normal saline

STEP 3. Cover the abbreviations with your hand and try to remember them.
STEP 4. Cover the terms and try to remember them.
STEP 5. Cover the entire list and try to write it on scrap paper.
STEP 6. Cover the top half of this page.

STEP 7. Take this check.

1. _____ nothing by mouth

2. **N/S** _____

3. **NG** _____

4. _____ negative

5. _____ newborn

STEP 8. Check your answers on the next page.

ANSWERS
1. **NPO**   Nothing by mouth
2. **N/S**   Normal saline
3. **NG**   Nasogastric
4. **neg**   Negative
5. **NB**   Newborn

If you did not get all of them correct, go back and practice STEPS 1 through 5. If you did, **VERY GOOD!** *Now continue.*

STEP 1. Study these abbreviations.

O₂   Oxygen
OB   Obstetrics
OD   Right eye
OPD   Outpatient department
os   Mouth

STEP 2. Cover the abbreviations with your hand and try to remember them.
STEP 3. Cover the terms and try to remember them.
STEP 4. Cover the entire list and try to write it on scrap paper.

STEP 5. Cover the bottom half of this page.
STEP 6. Take this check.

1. _____ right eye

2. _____ oxygen

3. **OPD** _____

4. _____ mouth

5. **OB** _____

STEP 7. Uncover the bottom half of this page and check your answers.

ANSWERS
1. **OD**   Right eye
2. **O₂**   Oxygen
3. **OPD**   Outpatient department
4. **os**   Mouth
5. **OB**   Obstetrics

*If you did not get all of them correct, go back and practice STEPS 1
through 4. If you did,* GOOD! *Now continue.*

STEP 1. Cover the bottom half of this page.
STEP 2. Study these abbreviations.

OS	Left eye
OU	Both eyes
oz, ʒ	Ounce
p̄	After
pc	After meals

STEP 3. Cover the abbreviations with your hand and try to remember them.
STEP 4. Cover the terms and try to remember them.
STEP 5. Cover the entire list and try to write it on scrap paper.
STEP 6. Cover the top half of this page.

STEP 7. Take this check.

1. _____ after

2. **pc** _____

3. _____ ounce

4. **OS** _____

5. _____ both eyes

STEP 8. Check your answers on the next page.

ANSWERS

1. p̄   After
2. **pc**   After meals
3. **oz, ʒ**   Ounce
4. **OS**   Left eye
5. **OU**   Both eyes

If you did not get all of them correct, review STEPS 1 through 5. If you did, GREAT! *Now continue.*

STEP 1. Study these abbreviations.

         ped   Pediatric
         PF   Pulmonary function
         PID   Pelvic inflammatory disease
         PM   Evening
         po   by mouth, orally

STEP 2. Cover the abbreviations with your hand and try to remember them.

STEP 3. Cover the terms and try to remember them.

STEP 4. Cover the entire list and try to write it on scrap paper.

STEP 5. Cover the bottom half of this page.
STEP 6. Take this check.

    1. _____ evening

    2. _____ pediatric

    3. **PF** _____

    4. _____ by mouth, orally

    5. **PID** _____

STEP 7. Uncover the bottom half of this page and check your answers.

ANSWERS

1. **PM**   Evening
2. **ped**   Pediatric
3. **PF**   Pulmonary function
4. **po**   By mouth, orally
5. **PID**   Pelvic inflammatory disease

If you did not get all of them correct, review STEPS 1 through 4. If you did, GOOD! *Continue.*

STEP 1. Cover the bottom half of this page.
STEP 2. Study these abbreviations.

PP	Postprandial
prn	Whenever necessary
pro time	Prothrombin time
pt	patient, pint
Px	Prognosis

STEP 3. Cover the abbreviations with your hand and try to remember them.
STEP 4. Cover the terms and try to remember them.
STEP 5. Cover the entire list and try to write it on scrap paper.
STEP 6. Cover the top half of this page.

STEP 7. Take this check.

1. _____ prothrombin time

2. **prn** _____

3. **Px** _____

4. _____ patient, pint

5. **PP** _____

STEP 8. Check your answers on the next page.

ANSWERS

1. **pro time** Prothrombin time
2. **prn** Whenever necessary
3. **Px** Prognosis
4. **pt** Patient, pint
5. **PP** Postprandial

If you did not get all of them correct, review STEPS 1 through 5. If you did, SUPER!

You have now learned 150 abbreviations. A review of the 150 abbreviations appears below and on the next pages.

STEP 1. Study the 150 abbreviations you should know.

1.	āā	Of each, equal parts
2.	abd	Abdomen
3.	ac	Before meals
4.	AD	Right ear
5.	ad lib	As desired
6.	adm	Admission
7.	AK	Above the knee
8.	AM	Morning
9.	amb	Ambulate
10.	amp	Ampule
11.	amt	Amount
12.	AP	Anteroposterior
13.	ARD	Acute respiratory distress
14.	AS	Left ear
15.	ASA	Aspirin
16.	as tol	As tolerated
17.	AV	Arteriovenous, atrioventricular
18.	ax	Axillary
19.	BaE	Barium enema
20.	bid	Twice a day
21.	BMR	Basal metabolic rate
22.	BP	Blood pressure
23.	BR	Bed rest
24.	BRP	Bathroom privileges
25.	BS	Blood sugar
26.	BT	Bleeding time
27.	BUN	Blood urea nitrogen
28.	Bx	Biopsy
29.	C	Centigrade
30.	c̄	With

31.	**CA**	Carcinoma
32.	**Ca^{++}**	Calcium
33.	**cap**	Capsule
34.	**cath**	Catheter
35.	**CBC**	Complete blood count
36.	**CC**	Chief complaint
37.	**CHD**	Congenital heart disease
38.	**chr**	Chronic
39.	**Cl**	Chloride
40.	**CNS**	Central nervous system
41.	**CO$_2$**	Carbon dioxide
42.	**COPD**	Chronic obstructive pulmonary disease
43.	**C-section**	Cesarean section
44.	**CSF**	Cerebrospinal fluid
45.	**cu mm**	Cubic millimeter
46.	**CVA**	Cerebrovascular accident
47.	**CXR**	Chest x-ray
48.	**cysto**	Cystoscopy
49.	**DAT**	Diet as tolerated
50.	**DC**	Discontinue
51.	**D & C**	Dilation and curettage
52.	**diag, Dx**	Diagnosis
53.	**diff**	Differential white blood count
54.	**DM**	Diabetes mellitus
55.	**DOB**	Date of birth
56.	**dr, 3**	Dram
57.	**DT**	Delirium tremens
58.	**DUB**	Dysfunctional uterine bleeding
59.	**EEG**	Electroencephalogram
60.	**EENT**	Eye, ear, nose, throat
61.	**EKG**	Electrocardiogram
62.	**elix**	Elixir
63.	**EMG**	Electromyogram
64.	**ER**	Emergency room
65.	**exc**	Excision
66.	**F**	Fahrenheit
67.	**FBS**	Fasting blood sugar
68.	**FDA**	Food and Drug Administration
69.	**Fe**	Iron
70.	**FH**	Family history
71.	**FHT**	Fetal heart tone
72.	**FSH**	Follicle-stimulating hormone
73.	**FUO**	Fever of undetermined origin
74.	**GB**	Gallbladder
75.	**GBS**	Gallbladder series
76.	**Gc**	Gonorrhea

77.	**GI**	Gastrointestinal
78.	**gm**	Gram
79.	**gr**	Grain
80.	**GTT**	Glucose tolerance test
81.	**gtt**	Drop
82.	**Gyn**	Gynecology
83.	**HCl**	Hydrochloric acid
84.	**Hct**	Hematocrit
85.	**Hgb**	Hemoglobin
86.	**H_2O**	Water
87.	**H_2O_2**	Hydrogen peroxide
88.	**H & P**	History and physical
89.	**hs**	Hour of sleep
90.	**HVD**	Hypertensive vascular disease
91.	**Hx**	History
92.	**hypo**	Hypodermic injection
93.	**I^{131}**	Radioactive iodine
94.	**IM**	Intramuscular
95.	**inf**	Infusion
96.	**inj**	Injection
97.	**IPPB**	Intermittent positive pressure breathing
98.	**IQ**	Intelligence quotient
99.	**IUD**	Intrauterine device
100.	**IV**	Intravenous
101.	**IVP**	Intravenous pyelogram
102.	**K^+**	Potassium
103.	**kg**	Kilogram
104.	**KUB**	Kidney, ureter, bladder
105.	**KVO**	Keep vein open
106.	**L**	Liter, left, lumbar spine
107.	**lab**	Laboratory
108.	**lb**	Pound
109.	**liq**	Liquid
110.	**LKS**	Liver, kidney, spleen
111.	**LLL**	Left lower lobe (lung)
112.	**LLQ**	Left lower quadrant (abd)
113.	**LMP**	Last menstrual period
114.	**LOC**	Level of consciousness
115.	**LUL**	Left upper lobe (lung)
116.	**LUQ**	Left upper quadrant (abd)
117.	**L & W**	Living and well
118.	**mEq**	Milliequivalent
119.	**Mg^{++}**	Magnesium
120.	**mg**	Milligram
121.	**MI**	Myocardial infarction
122.	**mm**	Millimeter

123. Mn^{--} Manganese
124. Na^+ Sodium
125. **NaCl**   Sodium chloride
126. **NB**   Newborn
127. **neg**   Negative
128. **NG**   Nasogastric
129. **NPO**   Nothing by mouth
130. **N/S**   Normal saline
131. O_2 Oxygen
132. **OB**   Obstetrics
133. **OD**   Right eye
134. **OPD**   Outpatient department
135. **os**   Mouth
136. **OS**   Left eye
137. **OU**   Both eyes
138. **oz, ʒ**   Ounce
139. **p̄**   After
140. **pc**   After meals
141. **ped**   Pediatric
142. **PF**   Pulmonary function
143. **PID**   Pelvic inflammatory disease
144. **PM**   Evening
145. **po**   By mouth, orally
146. **PP**   Postprandial
147. **prn**   Whenever necessary
148. **pro time** Prothrombin time
149. **pt**   Patient, pint
150. **Px**   Prognosis

STEP 2. Take this check.

1. **GL**_____

2. _____ mouth

3. **p̄** _____

4. _____ ounce

5. _____ twice a day

6. **lb** _____

7. **Px** _____

8. _____ milligram

9. **FSH** _____

10. _____ atrioventricular

11. **CSF** _____

12. **prn** _____

13. _____ cystoscopy

14. **OS** _____

15. **PF** _____

16. _____ oxygen

17. _____ grain

18. **PP** _____

19. _____ newborn

20. _____ by mouth, orally

21. _____ obstetrics

22. **hypo** _____

23. _____ potassium

24. **LUQ** _____

25. **GBS** _____

STEP 3. Check your answers on the next page.

ANSWERS

1. **GI** Gastrointestinal
2. **os** Mouth
3. **p̄** After
4. **oz, ʒ** Ounce
5. **bid** Twice a day
6. **lb** Pound
7. **Px** Prognosis
8. **mg** Milligram
9. **FSH** Follicle-stimulating hormone
10. **AV** Atrioventricular
11. **CSF** Cerebrospinal fluid
12. **prn** Whenever necessary
13. **cysto** Cystoscopy
14. **OS** Left eye
15. **PF** Pulmonary function
16. **O$_2$** Oxygen
17. **gr** Grain
18. **PP** Postprandial
19. **NB** Newborn
20. **po** By mouth, orally
21. **OB** Obstetrics
22. **hypo** Hypodermic injection
23. **K$^+$** Potassium
24. **LUQ** Left upper quadrant (abd)
25. **GBS** Gallbladder series

If you missed more than two, review STEP 1. You are getting very close to the end; keep up the good study habits. If you did not miss any, TERRIFIC! *Please continue.*

STEP 1. Cover the bottom half of this page.

STEP 2. Study these abbreviations.

qd	Daily
qh	Every hour
q3h	Every three hours
qid	Four times a day
qod	Every other day

STEP 3. Cover the abbreviations with your hand and try to remember them.

STEP 4. Cover the terms and try to remember them.

STEP 5. Cover the entire list and try to write it on scrap paper.

STEP 6. Cover the top half of this page.

STEP 7. Take this check.

1. **qod** _____

2. _____ daily

3. **q3h** _____

4. _____ four times a day

5. **qh** _____

STEP 8. Check your answers on the next page.

ANSWERS

1. **qod** Every other day
2. **qd** Daily
3. **q3h** Every three hours
4. **qid** Four times a day
5. **qh** Every hour

If you did not get them all correct, review STEPS 1 through 5. If you did, keep on going!

STEP 1. Study these abbreviations.

RBC	Red blood cell, red blood count
RLQ	Right lower quadrant (abd)
RO	Rule out
RUQ	Right upper quadrant (abd)
Rx	Therapy

STEP 2. Cover the abbreviations and try to remember them.
STEP 3. Cover the terms and try to remember them.
STEP 4. Cover the entire list and try to write it on scrap paper.

STEP 5. Cover the bottom half of this page.
STEP 6. Take this check.

      1. **RO** _____

      2. _____ therapy

      3. _____ red blood cell, red blood count

      4. **RUQ** _____

      5. **RLQ** _____

STEP 7. Uncover the bottom half of this page and check your answers.

ANSWERS

1. **RO** Rule out
2. **Rx** Therapy
3. **RBC** Red blood cell, red blood count
4. **RUQ** Right upper quadrant (abd)
5. **RLQ** Right lower quadrant (abd)

If you missed any, review STEPS 1 through 4. If not, GREAT! Continue.

STEP 1. Cover the bottom half of this page.

STEP 2. Study these abbreviations.

s̄	Without
SB	Stillborn
SC	Subcutaneously
SMR	Submucous resection
SOB	Shortness of breath

STEP 3. Cover the abbreviations with your hand and try to remember them.

STEP 4. Cover the terms and try to remember them.

STEP 5. Cover the entire list and try to write it on scrap paper.

STEP 6. Cover the top half of this page.

STEP 7. Take this check.

1. _____ subcutaneously

2. **SMR** _____

3. s̄ _____

4. _____ stillborn

5. **SOB** _____

STEP 8. Check your answers on the next page.

ANSWERS
1. **SC** Subcutaneously
2. **SMR** Submucous resection
3. **s̄** Without
4. **SB** Stillborn
5. **SOB** Shortness of breath

If you missed any, review STEPS 1 through 5. If not, go on.

STEP 1. Study these abbreviations.

sol	Solution
sp gr	Specific gravity
ss	Half
stat	Immediately
subling	Sublingual, under the tongue

STEP 2. Cover the terms with your hand and try to remember them.
STEP 3. Cover the abbreviations and try to remember them.
STEP 4. Cover the entire list and try to write it on scrap paper.

STEP 5. Cover the bottom half of this page.
STEP 6. Take this check.

1. **stat** _____

2. _____ under the tongue

3. **ss** _____

4. **sp gr** _____

5. _____ solution

STEP 7. Uncover the bottom half of this page and check your answers.
Rewrite the answers as you check them.

ANSWERS
1. **stat**   Immediately
2. **subling**   Under the tongue
3. **ss**   Half
4. **sp gr**   Specific gravity
5. **sol**   Solution

If you missed any, review STEPS 1 through 4. If not, GREAT. Continue.

STEP 1. Cover the bottom half of this page.
STEP 2. Study these abbreviations.

Sx, sympt	Symptoms
T	Temperature
tab	Tablet
TAH	Total abdominal hysterectomy
TB	Tuberculosis

STEP 3. Cover the terms and try to remember them.
STEP 4. Cover the abbreviations and try to remember them.
STEP 5. Cover the entire list and try to write it on scrap paper.
STEP 6. Cover the top half of this page.

STEP 7. Take this check.

1. _____ tablet

2. _____ tuberculosis

3. **TAH** _____

4. _____ temperature

5. **Sx** _____

STEP 8. Check your answers on the next page.

ANSWERS

Rewrite the words on scrap paper as you check your answers.

1. **tab**   tablet
2. **TB**   Tuberculosis
3. **TAH**   Total abdominal hysterectomy
4. **T**   Temperature
5. **Sx**   Symptoms

If you missed any, review STEPS 1 through 5. If you did not, please continue.

STEP 1. Study the 175 abbreviations you should know.

1.	**āā**	Of each, equal parts
2.	**abd**	Abdomen
3.	**ac**	Before meals
4.	**AD**	Right ear
5.	**ad lib**	As desired
6.	**adm**	Admission
7.	**AK**	Above the knee
8.	**AM**	Morning
9.	**amb**	Ambulate
10.	**amp**	Ampule
11.	**amt**	Amount
12.	**AP**	Anteroposterior
13.	**ARD**	Acute respiratory distress
14.	**AS**	Left ear
15.	**ASA**	Aspirin
16.	**as tol**	As tolerated
17.	**AV**	Arteriovenous, atrioventricular
18.	**ax**	Axillary
19.	**BaE**	Barium enema
20.	**bid**	Twice a day
21.	**BMR**	Basal metabolic rate
22.	**BP**	Blood pressure
23.	**BR**	Bed rest
24.	**BRP**	Bathroom privileges
25.	**BS**	Blood sugar
26.	**BT**	Bleeding time
27.	**BUN**	Blood urea nitrogen
28.	**Bx**	Biopsy
29.	**C**	Centigrade
30.	**c̄**	With
31.	**CA**	Carcinoma

32. Ca^{++} Calcium
33. cap   Capsule
34. cath   Catheter
35. CBC   Complete blood count
36. CC   Chief complaint
37. CHD   Congenital heart disease
38. chr   Chronic
39. Cl   Chloride
40. CNS   Central nervous system
41. CO_2 Carbon dioxide
42. COPD   Chronic obstructive pulmonary disease
43. C-section   Cesarean section
44. CSF   Cerebrospinal fluid
45. cu mm   Cubic millimeter
46. CVA   Cerebrovascular accident
47. CXR   Chest x-ray
48. cysto   Cystoscopy
49. DAT   Diet as tolerated
50. DC   Discontinue
51. D & C   Dilation and curettage
52. diag, Dx   Diagnosis
53. diff   Differential white blood count
54. DM   Diabetes mellitus
55. DOB   Date of birth
56. dr, ʒ   Dram
57. DT   Delirium tremens
58. DUB   Dysfunctional uterine bleeding
59. EEG   Electroencephalogram
60. EENT   Eye, ear, nose, throat
61. EKG   Electrocardiogram
62. elix   Elixir
63. EMG   Electromyogram
64. ER   Emergency room
65. exc   Excision
66. F   Fahrenheit
67. FBS   Fasting blood sugar
68. FDA   Food and Drug Administration
69. Fe   Iron
70. FH   Family history
71. FHT   Fetal heart tone
72. FSH   Follicle-stimulating hormone
73. FUO   Fever of undetermined origin
74. GB   Gallbladder
75. GBS   Gallbladder series
76. Gc   Gonorrhea
77. GI   Gastrointestinal

78.	**gm**	Gram
79.	**gr**	Grain
80.	**GTT**	Glucose tolerance test
81.	**gtt**	Drop
82.	**Gyn**	Gynecology
83.	**HCl**	Hydrochloric acid
84.	**Hct**	Hematocrit
85.	**Hgb**	Hemoglobin
86.	**H_2O**	Water
87.	**H_2O_2**	Hydrogen peroxide
88.	**H & P**	History and physical
89.	**hs**	Hour of sleep
90.	**HVD**	Hypertensive vascular disease
91.	**Hx**	History
92.	**hypo**	Hypodermic injection
93.	**I^{131}**	Radioactive iodine
94.	**IM**	Intramuscular
95.	**inf**	Infusion
96.	**inj**	Injection
97.	**IPPB**	Intermittent positive pressure breathing
98.	**IQ**	Intelligence quotient
99.	**IUD**	Intrauterine device
100.	**IV**	Intravenous
101.	**IVP**	Intravenous pyelogram
102.	**K^+**	Potassium
103.	**kg**	Kilogram
104.	**KUB**	Kidney, ureter, bladder
105.	**KVO**	Keep vein open
106.	**L**	Liter, left, lumbar spine
107.	**lab**	Laboratory
108.	**lb**	Pound
109.	**liq**	Liquid
110.	**LKS**	Liver, kidney, spleen
111.	**LLL**	Left lower lobe (lung)
112.	**LLQ**	Left lower quadrant (abd)
113.	**LMP**	Last menstrual period
114.	**LOC**	Level of consciousness
115.	**LUL**	Left upper lobe (lung)
116.	**LUQ**	Left upper quadrant (abd)
117.	**L & W**	Living and well
118.	**mEq**	Milliequivalent
119.	**Mg^{++}**	Magnesium
120.	**mg**	Milligram
121.	**MI**	Myocardial infarction
122.	**mm**	Millimeter
123.	**Mn^{--}**	Manganese

124.	Na^+	Sodium
125.	NaCl	Sodium chloride
126.	NB	Newborn
127.	neg	Negative
128.	NG	Nasogastric
129.	NPO	Nothing by mouth
130.	N/S	Normal saline
131.	O_2	Oxygen
132.	OB	Obstetrics
133.	OD	Right eye
134.	OPD	Outpatient department
135.	os	Mouth
136.	OS	Left eye
137.	OU	Both eyes
138.	oz, ʒ	Ounce
139.	p̄	After
140.	pc	After meals
141.	ped	Pediatric
142.	PF	Pulmonary function
143.	PID	Pelvic inflammatory disease
144.	PM	Evening
145.	po	By mouth, orally
146.	PP	Postprandial
147.	prn	Whenever necessary
148.	pro time	Prothrombin time
149.	pt	Patient, pint
150.	Px	Prognosis
151.	qd	Daily
152.	qh	Every hour
153.	q3h	Every three hours
154.	qid	Four times a day
155.	qod	Every other day
156.	RBC	Red blood cell, red blood count
157.	RLQ	Right lower quadrant (abd)
158.	RO	Rule out
159.	RUQ	Right upper quadrant (abd)
160.	Rx	Therapy
161.	s̄	Without
162.	SB	Stillborn
163.	SC	Subcutaneously
164.	SMR	Submucous resection
165.	SOB	Shortness of breath
166.	sol	Solution
167.	sp gr	Specific gravity
168.	ss	Half

169.	**stat**	Immediately
170.	**subling**	Sublingual, under the tongue
171.	**Sx, sympt**	Symptoms
172.	**T**	Temperature
173.	**tab**	Tablet
174.	**TAH**	Total abdominal hysterectomy
175.	**TB**	Tuberculosis

STEP 2. Take this check.

1. **pc** _____

2. _____ fever of undetermined origin

3. **NB** _____

4. _____ blood urea nitrogen

5. _____ lumbar spine

6. _____ four times a day

7. **OD** _____

8. _____ prognosis

9. **dr, ʒ** _____

10. _____ every hour

11. _____ ounce

12. **AD** _____

13. _____ red blood cell, red blood count

14. _____ potassium

15. _____ submucous resection

16. **hs** _____

17. _____ drop

18. **Rx** _____

19. _____ rule out

20. **ss** _____

21. **PF** _____

22. _____ tablet

23. _____ without

24. **Sx** _____

25. _____ both eyes

STEP 3. Check your answers on the next page.

ANSWERS

1. **pc**   After meals
2. **FUO**   Fever of undetermined origin
3. **NB**   Newborn
4. **BUN**   Blood urea nitrogen
5. **L**   Liter, left, lumbar spine
6. **qid**   Four times a day
7. **OD**   Right eye
8. **Px**   Prognosis
9. **dr, ʒ**   Dram
10. **qh**   Every hour
11. **oz, ʒ**   Ounce
12. **AD**   Right ear
13. **RBC**   Red blood cell, red blood count
14. **K⁺**   Potassium
15. **SMR**   Submucous resection
16. **hs**   Hour of sleep
17. **gtt**   Drop
18. **Rx**   Therapy
19. **RO**   Rule out
20. **ss**   Half
21. **PF**   Pulmonary function
22. **tab**   Tablet
23. **s̄**   Without
24. **Sx**   Symptom
25. **OU**   Both eyes

If you missed more than two, it is imperative that you go back and review the previous 175 abbreviations. Hang on, you are almost finished with this section of the book. If you did not miss any, GOOD! Now go on.

STEP 1. Cover the bottom half of this page.
STEP 2. Study these abbreviations.

tid	Three times a day
TUR	Transurethral resection
Tx	Treatment
UGI	Upper gastrointestinal
ung	Ointment

STEP 3. Cover the abbreviations and try to remember them.
STEP 4. Cover the terms and try to remember them.
STEP 5. Cover the entire list and try to write it on scrap paper.
STEP 6. Cover the top half of this page.

STEP 7. Take this check.

1. _____ treatment

2. _____ three times a day

3. **TUR** _____

4. **UGI** _____

5. _____ ointment

STEP 8. Check your answers on the next page.

ANSWERS

1. **Tx**   Treatment
2. **tid**   Three times a day
3. **TUR**   Transurethral resection
4. **UGI**   Upper gastrointestinal
5. **ung**   Ointment

If you did not get them all correct, review STEPS 1 through 5. If you did, go on.

STEP 1. Study these abbreviations.

URI	Upper respiratory infection
UTI	Urinary tract infection
VC	Vital capacity
VDRL	Venereal Disease Research Laboratories
VO	Verbal orders

STEP 2. Cover the abbreviations with your hand and try to remember them.
STEP 3. Cover the terms and try to remember them.
STEP 4. Cover the entire list and try to write it on scrap paper.

STEP 5. Cover the bottom half of this page.
STEP 6. Take this check.

1. _____ vital capacity

2. **VDRL** _____

3. _____ verbal orders

4. **UTI** _____

5. **URI** _____

STEP 7. Uncover the bottom half of this page and check your answers.

ANSWERS
1. **VC**   Vital capacity
2. **VDRL**   Venereal Disease Research Laboratories
3. **VO**   Verbal orders
4. **UTI**   Urinary tract infection
5. **URI**   Upper respiratory infection

If you missed any, review STEPS 1 through 4. If not, continue.

STEP 1. Cover the bottom half of this page. These are the last five abbreviations to be learned: you've made it!

STEP 2. Study these abbreviations.

VP   Venous pressure
WBC   White blood count, white blood cell
WF   White female
WM   White male
wt   Weight

STEP 3. For the last time, cover the abbreviations with your hand and try to remember them.

STEP 4. Cover the terms and try to remember them.

STEP 5. Cover the entire list and try to write it on scrap paper.

STEP 6. Cover the top half of this page.

STEP 7. Take this check.

1. **WF** _____

2. _____ weight

3. **VP** _____

4. _____ white blood count

5. **WM** _____

STEP 8. Check your answers on the next page.

ANSWERS
1. **WF** White female
2. **wt** Weight
3. **VP** Venous pressure
4. **WBC** White blood count
5. **WM** White male

If you did not get them all correct, review STEPS 1 through 5. If you did, CONGRATULATIONS! *Now just one more review.*

YOU HAVE NOW STUDIED AND LEARNED 190 ABBREVIATIONS. THE FOLLOWING IS A LIST OF ALL OF THESE. LOOK THEM OVER WELL BEFORE TAKING YOUR LAST REVIEW CHECK.

Study the 190 abbreviations you should know.

1.	**āā**	Of each, equal parts
2.	**abd**	Abdomen
3.	**ac**	Before meals
4.	**AD**	Right ear
5.	**ad lib**	As desired
6.	**adm**	Admission
7.	**AK**	Above the knee
8.	**AM**	Morning
9.	**amb**	Ambulate
10.	**amp**	Ampule
11.	**amt**	Amount
12.	**AP**	Anteroposterior
13.	**ARD**	Acute respiratory distress
14.	**AS**	Left ear
15.	**ASA**	Aspirin
16.	**as tol**	As tolerated
17.	**AV**	Arteriovenous, atrioventricular
18.	**ax**	Axillary
19.	**BaE**	Barium enema
20.	**bid**	Twice a day
21.	**BMR**	Basal metabolic rate
22.	**BP**	Blood pressure
23.	**BR**	Bed rest
24.	**BRP**	Bathroom privileges
25.	**BS**	Blood sugar
26.	**BT**	Bleeding time
27.	**BUN**	Blood urea nitrogen

c/o
complains

28.	**Bx**	Biopsy
29.	**C**	Centigrade
30.	**c̄**	With
31.	**CA**	Carcinoma
32.	**Ca⁺⁺**	Calcium
33.	**cap**	Capsule
34.	**cath**	Catheter
35.	**CBC**	Complete blood count
36.	**CC**	Chief complaint
37.	**CHD**	Congenital heart disease
38.	**chr**	Chronic
39.	**Cl**	Chloride
40.	**CNS**	Central nervous system
41.	**CO₂**	Carbon dioxide
42.	**COPD**	Chronic obstructive pulmonary disease
43.	**C-section**	Cesarean section
44.	**CSF**	Cerebrospinal fluid
45.	**cu mm**	Cubic millimeter
46.	**CVA**	Cerebrovascular accident
47.	**CXR**	Chest x-ray
48.	**cysto**	Cystoscopy
49.	**DAT**	Diet as tolerated
50.	**DC**	Discontinue or Discharge
51.	**D & C**	Dilation and curettage
52.	**diag, Dx**	Diagnosis
53.	**diff**	Differential white blood count
54.	**DM**	Diabetes mellitus
55.	**DOB**	Date of birth
56.	**dr, ʒ**	Dram
57.	**DT**	Delirium tremens
58.	**DUB**	Dysfunctional uterine bleeding
59.	**EEG**	Electroencephalogram
60.	**EENT**	Eye, ear, nose, throat
61.	**EKG**	Electrocardiogram
62.	**elix**	Elixir
63.	**EMG**	Electromyogram
64.	**ER**	Emergency room
65.	**exc**	Excision
66.	**F**	Fahrenheit
67.	**FBS**	Fasting blood sugar
68.	**FDA**	Food and Drug Administration
69.	**Fe**	Iron
70.	**FH**	Family history
71.	**FHT**	Fetal heart tone
72.	**FSH**	Follicle-stimulating hormone
73.	**FUO**	Fever of undetermined origin

74. **GB** — Gallbladder
75. **GBS** — Gallbladder series
76. **Gc** — Gonorrhea
77. **GI** — Gastrointestinal
78. **gm** — Gram
79. **gr** — Grain
80. **GTT** — Glucose tolerance test
81. **gtt** — Drop
82. **Gyn** — Gynecology
83. **HCl** — Hydrochloric acid
84. **Hct** — Hematocrit
85. **Hgb** — Hemoglobin
86. **H$_2$O** — Water
87. **H$_2$O$_2$** — Hydrogen peroxide
88. **H & P** — History and physical
89. **hs** — Hour of sleep
90. **HVD** — Hypertensive vascular disease
91. **Hx** — History
92. **hypo** — Hypodermic injection
93. **I^{131}** — Radioactive iodine
94. **IM** — Intramuscular
95. **inf** — Infusion
96. **inj** — Injection
97. **IPPB** — Intermittent positive pressure breathing
98. **IQ** — Intelligence quotient
99. **IUD** — Intrauterine device
100. **IV** — Intravenous
101. **IVP** — Intravenous pyelogram
102. **K$^+$** — Potassium
103. **kg** — Kilogram
104. **KUB** — Kidney, ureter, bladder
105. **KVO** — Keep vein open
106. **L** — Liter, left, lumbar spine
107. **lab** — Laboratory
108. **lb** — Pound
109. **liq** — Liquid
110. **LKS** — Liver, kidney, spleen
111. **LLL** — Left lower lobe (lung)
112. **LLQ** — Left lower quadrant (abd)
113. **LMP** — Last menstrual period
114. **LOC** — Level of consciousness *Loss g Consc*
115. **LUL** — Left upper lobe (lung)
116. **LUQ** — Left upper quadrant (abd)
117. **L & W** — Living and well
118. **mEq** — Milliequivalent
119. **Mg^{++}** — Magnesium

120.	**mg**	Milligram
121.	**MI**	Myocardial infarction
122.	**mm**	Millimeter *muscle*
123.	**Mn**⁻⁻	Manganese
124.	**Na**⁺	Sodium *Na⁺*
125.	**NaCl**	Sodium chloride
126.	**NB**	Newborn
127.	**neg**	Negative
128.	**NG**	Nasogastric
129.	**NPO**	Nothing by mouth
130.	**N/S**	Normal saline
131.	**O₂**	Oxygen
132.	**OB**	Obstetrics
133.	**OD**	Right eye
134.	**OPD**	Outpatient department
135.	**os**	Mouth
136.	**OS**	Left eye
137.	**OU**	Both eyes
138.	**oz, ʒ**	Ounce
139.	**p̄**	After
140.	**pc**	After meals
141.	**ped**	Pediatric
142.	**PF**	Pulmonary function
143.	**PID**	Pelvic inflammatory disease
144.	**PM**	Evening
145.	**po**	By mouth, orally
146.	**PP**	Postprandial
147.	**prn**	Whenever necessary
148.	**pro time**	Prothrombin time
149.	**pt**	Patient, pint
150.	**Px**	Prognosis
151.	**qd**	Daily
152.	**qh**	Every hour
153.	**q3h**	Every three hours
154.	**qid**	Four times a day
155.	**qod**	Every other day
156.	**RBC**	Red blood cell, red blood count
157.	**RLQ**	Right lower quadrant (abd)
158.	**RO**	Rule out
159.	**RUQ**	Right upper quadrant (abd)
160.	**Rx**	Therapy
161.	**s̄**	Without
162.	**SB**	Stillborn
163.	**SC**	Subcutaneously
164.	**SMR**	Submucous resection
165.	**SOB**	Shortness of breath

a: before

166.	**sol**	Solution
167.	**sp gr**	Specific gravity
168.	**ss**	Half
169.	**stat**	Immediately
170.	**subling**	Sublingual, under the tongue
171.	**Sx, sympt**	Symptoms
172.	**T**	Temperature
173.	**tab**	Tablet
174.	**TAH**	Total abdominal hysterectomy
175.	**TB**	Tuberculosis
176.	**tid**	Three times a day
177.	**TUR**	Transurethral resection
178.	**Tx**	Treatment
179.	**UGI**	Upper gastrointestinal
180.	**ung**	Ointment
181.	**URI**	Upper respiratory infection
182.	**UTI**	Urinary tract infection
183.	**VC**	Vital capacity
184.	**VDRL**	Venereal Disease Research Laboratories
185.	**VO**	Verbal orders
186.	**VP**	Venous pressure
187.	**WBC**	White blood count, white blood cell
188.	**WF**	White female
189.	**WM**	White male
190.	**wt**	Weight

MEDICAL ABBREVIATIONS REVIEW

Indicate the correct term or abbreviation for each of the following:

1. _____ sodium chloride

2. _____ half

3. HCL _____

4. abd _____

5. tid _____

6. _____ barium enema

7. _____ oxygen

8. os _____

9. _____ kilogram

10. _____ grain

11. Ca^{++} _____

12. Tx _____

13. ung _____

14. CSF _____

15. _____ by mouth

16. _____ radioactive iodine

17. _____ milliequivalent

18. N/S _____

19. _____ after

20. K^+ _____

21. ARD _____

22. IVP _____

23. āā _____

24. inf _____

25. _____ chronic

26. EKG _____

27. ad lib _____

28. **prn** _____

29. _____ after meals

30. _____ electromyogram

Check your answers on the following page. If you missed more than two, go back and study the final list of abbreviations.

GO TO THE INSTRUCTOR AND ASK FOR TEST NUMBER 9. IT WILL COVER ONLY ABBREVIATIONS. REMEMBER, YOU MUST ACHIEVE 80% MASTERY TO PASS.

ANSWERS

1. **NaCl**
2. **ss**
3. hydrochloric acid
4. abdomen
5. three times a day
6. **BaE**
7. **O$_2$**
8. mouth
9. **kg**
10. **gr**
11. calcium
12. treatment
13. ointment
14. cerebrospinal fluid
15. **po**
16. **I^{131}**
17. **mEq**
18. normal saline
19. **p̄**
20. potassium
21. acute respiratory distress
22. intravenous pyelogram
23. of each, equal parts
24. infusion
25. **chr**
26. electrocardiogram
27. as desired
28. whenever necessary
29. **pc**
30. **EMG**

FINAL REVIEW

Along with reviewing the entire programmed text, the following pages will help you prepare for the final examination.

Any information in this text may be used as test material for the final examination. Please remember, you must achieve at least 80% mastery to pass.

SUFFIXES

A suffix is a word ending that changes the meaning of the word root. Match the following suffixes with their correct meanings:

1. -spasm _____		a. hernia, protrusion
2. -itis _____		b. pain
3. -ectomy _____		c. surgical correction
4. -algia _____		d. fixation
5. -oma _____		e. suspension
6. -plasty _____		f. involuntary contraction
7. -pnea _____		g. disease
8. -desis _____		h. removal of, excision
9. -cele _____		i. to make a more or less permanent opening
10. -pexy _____		j. inflammation
11. -pathy _____		k. breathing
12. -lithotomy _____		l. cell
13. -cyte _____		m. development
14. -trophy _____		n. incision for removal of stones
15. -stomy _____		o. tumor

PREFIXES

Prefixes are word beginnings that give the proximity to or amount of the word root. Match the following prefixes:

1. circum- ____   a. four

2. trans- ____   b. under

3. extra- ____   c. through

4. intro- ____   d. two

5. multi- ____   e. against

6. quad- ____   f. near, toward

7. tachy- ____   g. into, in

8. hypo- ____   h. rapid

9. endo- ____   i. equal

10. bi- ____   j. around

11. equi- ____   k. with, joined

12. anti- ____   l. many

13. co-, con- ____   m. around

14. peri- ____   n. within

15. ad- ____   o. outside, beyond

WORD ROOTS

A word root is the foundation of the word. Define the following:

1. ilio _____
2. cardio _____
3. neuro _____
4. costo _____
5. chondro _____
6. salpingo _____
7. broncho _____
8. dermo _____
9. denti _____
10. ano _____

Give the word roots for the following:

11. ileum _____
12. small bowel _____
13. breast _____
14. skull _____
15. tongue _____
16. abdomen _____
17. bladder _____
18. prostate _____
19. muscle _____
20. mouth _____

Break down the following compound words and give their meanings.

1. jejunoileostomy

2. nephroureterolithiasis

3. left pneumobronchectomy

BASIC ANATOMY AND PHYSIOLOGY

Answer each question.

1. Name the four body cavities.
   a.
   b.
   c.
   d.

2. The largest of the body cavities is the _____.

3. Name the eight body systems.
   a.
   b.
   c.
   d.
   e.
   f.
   g.
   h.

Fill in the blank.

4. A word that means something out of the ordinary is_____.

5. If the problem was present at birth, it is said to be_____.

6. His blue eyes were transmitted from his parents; they were

   _____.

7. The age at which the reproductive organs become active is

   _____.

8. If the tumor is cancerous, it is _____.

9. The outcome of a disease is called the _____.

10. The pneumonia has been of long duration; it is _____.

11. If the tumor will not come back and is essentially harmless, it is

    called _____.

MUSCULAR AND SKELETAL SYSTEMS

Answer the following questions:

1. Bones that are around the middle of the body and act as protective shields are _____.

2. List four functions of the skeletal system.
   a.
   b.
   c.
   d.

3. In what part(s) of the body does one find long bones?

4. What is another name for long bones?

5. What is an example of an irregular joint?

6. What are the three different types of muscles?
   a.
   b.
   c.

7. The shoulder and hip are examples of what kind of joint?

8. What is the body doing when in the following positions?

   a. abducting an arm _____

   b. supine _____

   c. reaching inferiorly _____

   d. moving an arm medially _____

   e. prone _____

Unscramble the following terms:

9. foot bones
   (ttmaarssue)   _____

10. pertains to an erect position
    (thtoociarts)   _____

11. back of the head
    (coupcit)   _____

12. artificial replacement
    (ssrpheisot)   _____

13. paralysis of the legs
    (apapirglae)   _____

14. inner portion of an organ
    (lulmdae)   _____

15. kneecap
    (elapalt)   _____

16. sole of the foot
    (aplatrn)   _____

CIRCULATORY SYSTEM

Fill in the blank.

1. The cardiac muscle is a _____, _____ muscle.

2. The blood is made up of a liquid and solid part; of the two, which has the larger volume? _____

3. When one has too many white blood cells, they may have a disease called _____.

Match the following terms:

4. embolus ____   a. formation of a clot in blood vessel

5. ischemia ____   b. carries blood toward the heart

6. bradycardia ____   c. chamber or cavity

7. vein ____   d. white blood cell

8. myocardium ____   e. clot of air or blood

9. hemoglobin ____   f. profuse bleeding

10. atrium ____   g. pointed end of conical shape

11. thrombosis ____   h. muscle of the heart

12. angina ____   i. extremely high blood pressure

13. plasma ____   j. slow heartbeat

14. hemorrhage ____   k. carries blood away from the heart

15. leukocyte ____   l. one type of white blood cell

16. artery ____   m. temporary lack of blood supply

17. lymphocyte ____   n. liquid part of blood

18. hypertension ____   o. pain and oppressive feeling in the chest

19. apex ____   p. iron-containing pigment in red blood cells

RESPIRATORY SYSTEM

Fill in the blanks.

1. A waste product of the body's cells is _____.

2. The large muscle that separates the thoracic from the abdominopelvic cavity is the _____.

3. What functions does the respiratory system provide for the body?
   a.
   b.
   c.

4. Oxygenated blood is what color? (Bright or dark red.)

Select the correct medical term.

eupnea   naris
bronchus   hemoptysis
asphyxia   apnea
dyspnea   anoxia

5. _____ difficult or labored breathing

6. _____ nostril

7. _____ coughing up of blood

8. _____ branch of the trachea

9. _____ normal breathing

10. _____ temporary cessation of breathing

11. _____ deficient oxygen to supply tissues

URINARY SYSTEM

Fill in the blank.

1. When one is unable to retain discharges one is _____.

2. If swelling of the ankles is called _____.

3. If the urine sample was found to have too much sugar in it the patient has _____.

4. A rubber tube inserted into the bladder for elimination of urine is a

   _____.

5. The presence of pus in the urine is called _____.

6. A term referring to kidneys is _____.

7. Blood found in the urine is called _____.

8. When one wets the bed, it is called _____.

DIGESTIVE SYSTEM

Answer the following questions:

1. List the route that food takes through the body.
   a.
   b.
   c.
   d.
   e.
   f.
   g.

2. There are both mechanical and _____ processes in the breakdown of food.

Fill in the correct term.

edentia	anorexia	jaundice
singultus	caries	dehydration
hematemesis	enteritis	cachexia
gingivitis	peristalsis	eructation

3. _____ loss of appetite

4. _____ yellowness of skin

5. _____ blood in vomitus

6. _____ inflammation of gums

7. _____ decay of teeth

8. _____ hiccups

9. _____ ill health due to malnutrition

10. _____ inflammation of the intestines

11. _____ belching

12. _____ without teeth

REPRODUCTIVE SYSTEM

Answer the following questions:

1. What are the main purposes of the reproductive system?
   a.
   b.
   c.

2. Name the main organs of the female reproductive system.
   a.
   b.
   c.
   d.
   e.

3. Name the main organs of the male reproductive system.
   a.
   b.
   c.
   d.

Circle the correct spelling and give the definition.

4. AMENOREHA   AMMENORHEA   AMENORRHEA

   _____

5. EMBRYO   EMBRIO   EMBREO

   _____

6. LACTATION   LACETION   LACETATION

   _____

7. UMBILLICUS   UMBELICUS   UMBILICUS

   _____

8. ECTOPIT   ECTOPIC   ACTOPIC

   _____

NERVOUS SYSTEM

Answer these questions.

1. Name the three parts of the nervous system.
   a.
   b.
   c.

2. Because these structures are essential to life, nature has provided them extra padding and protection. Name these protective structures.
   a.
   b.

Match each term to its correct meaning.

3. paroxysm _____   a. fainting

4. cephalalgia _____   b. mental dullness or drowsiness

5. aphasia _____   c. dizziness

6. syncope _____   d. inability to express oneself

7. vertigo _____   e. convulsion

8. incoherence _____   f. loss of verbal comprehension

9. lethargic _____   g. headache

Define the following terms:

10. urticaria _____

11. epistaxis _____

12. lacrimal _____

13. diffuse _____

14. acidosis _____

15. cerumen _____

ANSWERS

Section 1

Page 3
1. b 2. a 3. c 4. c 5. b

Section 2

Page 6
1. **-centesis** Puncture
2. **-ectomy** Excision, removal
3. **-itis** Inflammation
4. **-scopy** Visualization, inspection
5. **-algia** Pain

Page 9
1. e 2. g 3. f 4. d 5. h 6. b 7. a 8. c

Page 12
1. e 2. g 3. h 4. f 5. a 6. b 7. d 8. c

Section 3

Page 14
1. **circum-** Around
2. **hypo-** Below
3. **trans-** Through
4. **post-** Behind, after
5. **multi-** Many

Page 16
Prefixes: 1. c 2. e or h 3. f 4. b 5. g 6. i 7. d 8. a 9. h or e
Suffixes: 1. b 2. c 3. d 4. a 5. e

Page 18
Prefixes: 1. j or g 2. h 3. b 4. d 5. f 6. i 7. c 8. g or j 9. e 10. a
Suffixes: 1. d 2. c 3. a 4. b 5. e

Page 20
Prefixes: 1. e 2. d 3. f 4. g 5. h 6. b 7. a 8. c
Suffixes: 1. d 2. c 3. b 4. a 5. e

Section 4

Page 24
Meaning: 1. pelvis of kidney 2. chest 3. spinal cord or bone marrow 4. head 5. thyroid gland 6. bladder 7. testicles
Word roots: 1. laparo 2. osteo 3. arterio 4. rhino, naso 5. myo 6. prostato 7. stomato

Page 28
Meaning: 1. teeth 2. skin 3. ovary 4. ileum 5. air 6. uterus 7. bronchus 8. ear
Word roots: 1. cranio 2. ophthalmo, oculo 3. glosso 4. masto 5. entero 6. cholecysto 7. appendico 8. ano

Page 32
1. before the thyroid 2. around the thyroid 3. through the thyroid 4. outside the thyroid 5. within the thyroid 6. under the thyroid 7. beside the thyroid 8. above the thyroid 9. many thyroid glands 10. excessive amount of thyroid

Section 5

Pages 33–34
1. a. word root b. prefix c. suffix 2. bronch/o 3. True 4. True 5. a. P b. S c. P d. P e. S f. P g. S h. P i. P j. S 6. a rib b. heart c. nerve d. liver 7. a. oophor b. oto c. dermo d. salpingo 8. a. If a suffix begins with a consonant, just add it to the root. b. If a suffix begins with a vowel, drop the vowel of the root and add the suffix. 9. For the suffixes -rhexis and -rhaphy, double the "r" and add it to the word root.

Page 39
1. opening between the fallopian tube and ureter 2. disorder of the skin with nervous tissue involvement 3. removal of kidney and ureter 4. inflammation of the kidney and bladder 5. removal of the ovary and fallopian tube 6. incision into the gallbladder and bowel

Section 6

Page 44
1. b 2. c 3. true 4. eight

Page 46
1. c 2. e 3. d 4. a 5. b 6. brachial 7. inguinal 8. carcinoma

Page 48
1. c 2. a 3. b 4. e 5. d 6. palliative—offering temporary relief 7. moribund—in a dying condition 8. syndrome—a set of symptoms that occur together 9. True 10. False 11. False

Section 7

Page 54
1. True 2. False 3. True 4. False 5. True 6. Supports, anchors, shapes, makes blood cells, protects, stores calcium 7. cartilage 8. short

Page 56
1. smooth, involuntary 2. cardiac 3. voluntary 4. warmth, strength 5. one-half, 40 to 50% 6. bones 7. taper, thin

Page 60
1. ball and socket 2. bones 3. ligaments 4. extension 5. flexion 6. articulation 7. proximal 8. lateral 9. supine 10. superior 11. posterior 12. abduct

Page 62
1. f 2. c 3. a 4. e 5. d 6. b 7. acetabulum 8. carpal 9. claudication 10. ambulatory

Page 64
1. membrane 2. occiput 3. plantar 4. medulla 5. phalanges 6. patella 7. metacarpus 8. artificial replacement 9. paralysis of the legs 10. middle section of the thoracic cavity

Page 65
1. pain in a bone 2. incision into the articular end of a bone 3. osteitis 4. congestion of blood in a bone 5. degenerative disease of bone joints 6. osteocephaloma 7. inflammation of bone and cartilage 8. defective bone development 9. resembling a bone 10. osteomalacia 11. tumor containing muscular and fibrous tissue 12. myocyte 13. formation of muscular tissue 14. fatty degeneration with destruction to muscle tissue 15. inflammation of cardiac muscle 16. myorrhexis 17. myosalpingitis 18. visualization of a joint with an arthroscope 19. arthrosis 20. arthrocele 21. surgical fixation of a joint

Section 8

Page 69
1. heart 2. striated, involuntary 3. a. carry oxygen and food to cells b. exchange oxygen and food for waste products c. carry waste to elimination points 4. anemia 5. phagocytosis

Page 73
1. capillary 2. antigen 3. apex 4. bradycardia 5. aneurysm 6. angina 7. embolus

Pages 75–76
1. d 2. g 3. e 4. b 5. f 6. a 7. c 8. hardening of the arteries 9. recording of an artery 10. subclavian artery 11. removal of inside of carotid artery 12. inner portion of an artery 13. blood clots in the vein 14. phlebitis 15. weakening in wall of an artery, causing a ballooning out 16. diseased heart muscle; heart attack 17. record or examination of blood or lymph vessels 18. myocarditis 19. pain in the heart 20. softening of the heart 21. cardiotomy 22. rupture of a vein

Page 82
1. d 2. h 3. b 4. j 5. i 6. a 7. c 8. f 9. g 10. e

Page 83
1. inflammation of nose 2. pneumonectomy 3. abnormal expansion of the bronchus of the lungs 4. bronchogenic 5. puncture into the chest cavity 6. x-ray of bronchus 7. pneumonitis 8. tracheotomy 9. esophagoscopy 10. softening of the rings of the trachea

Anatomy and Physiology Mid-review Answers

1. thoracic, spinal, cranial, abdominopelvic 2. cell 3. three of the following: supports, shapes, protects, anchors muscles, stores calcium, makes blood cells 4. cranium 5. any of the following: rib, breastbone (sternum), skull, backbone (vertebrae) 6. three of the following: long, flat, short, irregular 7. involuntary 8. striated, involuntary 9. anemic 10. artery 11. hinge 12. adduction 13. bradycardia 14. precordial 15. inhalation 16. exhalation 17. diaphragm 18. anoxia

Spelling and definition
1. **etiology**   Study of the causes of diseases
2. **syndrome**   A set of symptoms that occur together
3. **acetabulum**   Socket in the hip bone into which the head of the femur fits
4. **loin**   Area of the back between ribs and hip

5. **peripheral**   Pertaining to an outside surface
6. **diastole**   Relaxation of the heart
7. **aneurysm**   Weakening of the wall of an artery
8. **ischemia**   Temporary lack of blood supply to an area
9. **hemoptysis**   Coughing up of blood
10. **orthopnea**   Inability to breathe while lying down

Matching

1. b 2. c 3. e 4. g 5. f 6. d 7. a

Unscramble

1. thrombosis 2. leukocyte 3. vasospasm 4. hypertension 5. pulmonary

Section 9

Pages 90–91
1. excretory 2. kidneys 3. ureters 4. bladder 5. urethra 6. f 7. d 8. c 9. g 10. b
11. a 12. e 13. cystitis 14. incision into ureter to remove stones 15. pyelonephritis
16. making an opening into a ureter 17. renal hernia 18. suturing up a kidney 19.
cystoptosis

Section 10

Page 96
1. a. gastrointestinal tract
   b. alimentary canal
2. a. mechanical breakdown of food and chemicals
   b. absorption of nutrients into the circulatory system
3. digestive juices from the stomach, gallbladder, liver, and pancreas

Page 98
1. caries 2. cachexia 3. defecation 4. dehydration 5. anorexia 6. emesis 7. edentia 8. colic

Page 100
1. **glossal**   Pertaining to the tongue
2. **jaundice**   Yellow discoloration of skin
3. **hematemesis**   Blood in vomitus
4. **singultus**   Hiccups
5. **peristalsis**   Wavelike movement in digestive tract

Pages 100–101
6. gingivitis 7. flatus 8. paroxia 9. obese 10. palate 11. gastrectomy 12. colostomy
13. inflammation of the intestine 14. making an incision into the bile duct 15.
hernia of the intestine 16. gastrostomy 17. uncontrollable contraction of the
esophagus 18. esophagoscopy 19. enlargement of the liver 20. epigastrocele 21.
cholelithiasis 22. tumor of the mouth 23. visualization of the rectum with a scope

Section 11

Page 107
1. e 2. c 3. b 4. f 5. g 6. d 7. a 8. hysterectomy 9. orchioptosis 10. hysteroplasty 11. vasectomy 12. pain in the ovary 13. suspension of the uterus 14. right salpingooophorectomy

Section 12

Page 115
1. cephalalgia 2. hydrocephalus 3. psychosomatic 4. incoherence 5. vertigo 6. hormones 7. pituitary 8. vertebral column 9. any two of these: control consciousness; control mental processes; regulate body movements, functions 10. cranial, spinal, automatic 11. a. sympathetic fibers

Section 13

Page 118
1. afebrile 2. to remove by suction 3. cerumen 4. localized collection of pus in a cavity 5. amblyopia 6. section of tissue removed from a living specimen 7. cataract 8. serous fluid in the peritoneal cavity

Page 120
1. f 2. i 3. a 4. l 5. j 6. c 7. b 8. d 9. g 10. e 11. h 12. k

Page 122
1. pyrexia 2. photophobia 3. epistaxis 4. diplopia 5. urticaria 6. ulcer 7. stenosis 8. myopia 9. purulent

Final Review

Suffixes
1. f 2. j 3. h 4. b 5. o 6. c 7. k 8. d 9. a 10. e 11. g 12. n 13. l 14. m 15. i
Prefixes
1. j 2. c, m 3. o 4. g 5. l 6. a 7. h 8. b 9. n 10. d 11. i 12. e 13. k 14. c, m 15. f

Word Roots
1. bone 2. heart 3. nerve 4. rib 5. cartilage 6. fallopian tube 7. bronchus 8. skin 9. teeth 10. anus 11. ileo 12. entero 13. masto 14. cranio 15. glosso 16. laparo 17. cysto 18. prostato 19. myo 20. stomato

Compound Words
1. jejuno—jejunum, ileo—ileum, stomy—more or less permanent opening: making a more or less permanent opening between the jejunum and ileum of the bowel
2. nephro—kidneys, uretero—ureter, -lithiasis—removal of stones: removal of stones from the kidneys or ureter
3. pneumo—lung, broncho—bronchus, -ectomy—removal of: removal of left lung and bronchus

Basic Anatomy and Physiology
1. a. thoracic b. abdominopelvic c. cranial d. spinal 2. abdominopelvic 3. a. digestive b. respiratory c. urinary d. reproductive e. circulatory f. skeletal and muscular g. nervous h. endocrine 4. anomaly 5. congenital 6. inherited 7. puberty 8. malignant 9. prognosis 10. chronic 11. benign

Muscular and Skeletal Systems
1. axial 2. four of the following: supports, shapes, protects, makes blood cells, stores calcium, provides anchors for muscles 3. legs, toes, arms, fingers 4. appendicular 5. vertebrae 6. a. voluntary, smooth b. involuntary, striated c. smooth, cardiac, involuntary 7. ball and socket 8. a. moving an arm away from the body b. lying face up c. reaching toward the feet d. moving an arm toward the middle of the body e. lying face down 9. metatarsus 10. orthostatic 11. occiput 12. prosthesis 13. paraplegia 14. medulla 15. patella 16. plantar

Circulatory System
1. striated, involuntary 2. liquid 3. leukemia 4. e 5. m 6. j 7. b 8. h 9. p 10. c 11. a 12. o 13. n 14. f 15. d 16. k 17. l 18. i 19. g

Respiratory System
1. carbon dioxide (CO_2) 2. diaphragm 3. three of the following: aids in production of sound, eliminates waste, eliminates excess heat, provides exchange of gases between body and its environment 4. bright 5. dyspnea 6. naris 7. hemoptysis 8. bronchus 9. eupnea 10. apnea 11. anoxia

Urinary System
1. incontinent 2. edema 3. glycosuria 4. catheter 5. pyuria 6. renal 7. hematuria 8. enuresis

Digestive System
1. a. mouth b. pharynx c. esophagus d. stomach e. small bowel f. colon g. rectum to the anus 2. chemical 3. anorexia 4. jaundice 5. hematemesis 6. gingivitis 7. caries 8. singultus 9. cachexia 10. enteritis 11. eructation 12. edentia

Reproductive System
1. a. renewal of life b. sexual gratification c. hormonal secretion 2. a. mammary glands, breast b. two ovaries c. two fallopian tubes d. uterus e. vagina 3. a. scrotum b. penis c. testes d. duct system
4. **amenorrhea** Absence of menstrual flow
5. **embryo** Fetal development between second and eighth week
6. **lactation** Mammary glands secreting milk
7. **umbilicus** Naval; cord attaching fetus to mother
8. **ectopic** Implantation of fertile egg outside the uterus

Nervous System
1. a. brain b. spinal cord c. nerves 2. a. skull b. vertebral column 3. e 4. g 5. f 6. a 7. c 8. d 9. b 10. hives 11. nosebleed 12. pertaining to tears 13. widely scattered 14. condition in which there is an excessive amount of acid in the blood 15. earwax

RECOMMENDED REFERENCE BOOKS

For further information on either medical terms or anatomy and physiology, the following books will be helpful:

Anthony, C. P., and Alyn, I. B. *Structure and Function of the Body* (5th ed.). St. Louis: Mosby, 1976.

Birmingham, J. J. *Medical Terminology—A Self-Learning Module.* New York: McGraw-Hill, 1981.

Chabner, D. E. *The Language of Medicine: A Write-in Text Explaining Medical Terms* (2nd ed.). Philadelphia: Saunders, 1981.

Squires, B. P. *Basic Terms of Anatomy and Physiology.* Philadelphia: Saunders, 1970.

Thomas, C. L. (Ed.). *Taber's Cyclopedic Medical Dictionary* (14th ed.). Philadelphia: Davis, 1981.

INDEX

Abdomen, 61
Abdominopelvic, 41
Abduct, 58
Abnormal, 117
Abscess, 117
Acetabulum, 61
Acidosis, 117
Acute, 117
Adduct, 58
Adolescence, 106
Adrenal, 109
Afebrile, 117
Alignment, 61
Alkalosis, 117
Alveoli, 80
Amblyopia, 117
Ambulatory, 61
Amenorrhea, 106
Anastomosis, 97
Anemia, 67, 72
Aneurysm, 72
Angina, 72
Angioma, 72
Anomaly, 45
Anorexia, 97
Anoxia, 80
Anterior, 58
Antibody, 72
Anticoagulant, 68
Antigen, 72
Anus, 97
Aorta, 71
Apex, 72
Aphasia, 114
Apnea, 80
Appendectomy, 97
Appendicular, 49
Artery, 70, 72
Articulation, 57
Ascites, 117
Asepsis, 117
Asphyxia, 80
Aspirate, 117
Ataxia, 61
Atrium, 72
Atrophy, 61
Autopsy, 117
Axial, 49
Axilla, 117

Benign, 45
Biopsy, 117
Bladder, 87, 88, 89
Blood, 67
Bones, 52

flat, 52
irregular, 52
long, 52
short, 52
Brachial, 45
Bradycardia, 72
Bronchus, 80
Buttocks, 61

Cachexia, 97
Calculus, 97
Capillary, 72
Carcinoma, 45
Cardiac, 72
Caries, 97
Carpal, 61
Cataract, 117
Catheter, 89
Cephalalgia, 114
Cerebellum, 111, 112
Cerebrum, 111, 112
Cerumen, 117
Cervical, 61
Cholecystitis, 97
Cholesterol, 117
Chronic, 45
Circulatory, 67
Claudication, 61
Colic, 97
Colon, 97
Coma, 114
Congenital, 45
Cortex, 88, 89, 109
Costal, 61
Cranial cavity, 41
Crepitus, 97
Cutaneous, 45
Cyanosis, 80
Cytology, 45

Decubitus, 119
Defecation, 97
Dehydration, 97
Diaphoresis, 119
Diaphragm, 77, 78, 79, 80
Diastole, 72
Diffuse, 119
Digestive system, 93, 94
Diplopia, 119
Distal, 58
Dorsal, 58
Dysmenorrhea, 106
Dysphagia, 97
Dyspnea, 80
Dysuria, 89